You're Not Crazy!
An Overcomer's Guide
To Fibromyalgia

By
Dr. Timothy Weir, D.C.

Author: Dr. Timothy Weir
ISBN Number: 978-1-4303-1347-2
Copyright © 2010 by Dr. Timothy Weir.
Publisher: Lulu

DEDICATION

To my lovely wife, Rose. This book was her
idea. Her presence in my life has been a major
source of the healing presence that works in me.

Acknowledgments

I would like to take a moment and express deep gratitude to the many people in my life with whom I have worked to bring me to the point of writing a book.

To Rose Weir, my wife, partner in business and life, and my best friend. Without her intensity, love for me, love for business and life, this book would not be here. She is the one who said to me in the car one day, "why don't you write a book on FMS", and so here we are.

To Wendi, Nikki and Tyler and Alon, my four children.   These are the four greatest children in the world. I am truly blessed.   I am also blessed with two great son-in-laws, David Colgan and Michael Davis.

To my mother, Ione Weir, who gave me the understanding that you can do anything that you put your mind to, Thanks.   Her desire for creative writing gave me the desire to write this book.

To my dad, Julius, who is looking over from the portals of heaven, thanks for having been a great dad.   You instilled in me a zest for life.

To my brother, Dr. J. Michael Weir, you are the greatest brother in the world. You herded me into the direction of where I am now. I am grateful. Your wisdom has saved me much sorrow through the years.

In honor of my brother, Dr. Kevin Weir, who passed from this life in 2003. He was my school buddy, a great friend and a hero. He has left behind a legacy in his son, Dr. Mike Weir…carry on .

All the great motivators in my life, Doug Wead, Bob Proctor, Dr. Mark Chironna, Dr. Steve Lund, Dr. Steven Conway, and a host of others….Thank you.

Finally, I remember Karen Paine, M.D., my friend, coworker and incredible physician who passed away on July 18, 2007. As I sat with her the last couple of nights of her life as Karen Paine, it became ever so clear that you have close to 70 years to make a mark on the world…she did! Thanks Karen for all you did!

And finally, to you the readers who purchased this book.

Thank you all.

CONTENTS

IMPORTANT INFORMATION FOR THE READER

The information presented in this book has been compiled from my clinical experience and literary research. It is offered as a view of the relationship with the body, the mind, and the spirit and FMS. This book is not a vehicle for, nor is it intended for, self diagnosis or treatment of disease, nor is it a substitute for the advice and care of a licensed health care provider. This book is intended solely to help you make better judgments concerning your long-term health goals, and is not intended for the treatment of specific illnesses. No guarantee or assurance is given to anyone as to the specific results that may be obtained. If you are experiencing health problems, you should consult your doctor immediately. Remember, early examination and detection are important to successful treatment of FMS.

Dr. Timothy Weir, D.C.

Foreword

Chronic Fibromyalgia is one of those elusive conditions that are difficult to detect at first glance and perhaps even more difficult to diagnose, let alone treat. In a day and time when modern medicine has worked miracles in so many areas, treatment have proven to fall short in a full promise of recovery. The limitations of many of our medical approaches to the healing of the body have gone unquestioned until recently. Chronic sufferers have often found themselves going down long and winding dead end roads to misdiagnosis, and trial and error approaches to healing. Sometimes the attempted cures have been as painful as the condition itself. Given the fact that it is difficult to detect if one does not know what they are looking for or seeing, there is a breeding ground present for spending great amounts of money on treatments that will not improve the quality of one's life. Running from place to place, and clinic to clinic in hopes for a cure can lead to a great deal of darkness and despair.

Yet in the darkness a light is already shining. There is a rising generation of health care practitioners who are seeing a larger picture and treating a whole person. Dr. Tim Weir is one of an emerging and new breed of cutting edge healthcare professionals who has dedicated his life to the healing of persons. You can't be around him for any length of time and not sense his deep commitment to seeing people made whole and having a richer and fuller total life experience. His years in the practice of health care have afforded him the opportunity to touch thousands of lives and get the heart and soul of assisting individuals in cooperating with their bodies and attaining a greater degree of health and well being. He has had first hand experience with the sufferers of this strange condition and has seen the devastation it creates. In an effort to alleviate and ease the pain he has made room in his life to discover the missing pieces between what has been known and what has been unknown about this medical challenge. In the process he has found a beam of hope and has had wonderful results that have made a difference in the lives of many. You may be one of those silent sufferers who have cried out in desperation for an answer to your chronic condition. I believe Providence has led you to this little book to serve you in reclaiming your total health and well being and set you on the road to recovery. While you are reading a book about a medical condition, it won't read like one. It reads like a story of your life. Dr. Weir connects with you where you are and leads you gently and carefully on this seemingly dark path to a place where the light of hope is shining brightly. You will find yourself on page after page being able to identify with what is there. The reason is simple, Dr. Weir has one ultimate objective: to see you whole. Because he does his best to identify with you, in his writing you will immediately connect with him and build a therapeutic relationship. Dr. Weir will become as real to you in the pages of this book as he is to his patients in his own practice. His warmth and his light hearted approach to a very delicate challenge will both hold your interest and lay the foundation and groundwork for healing presence to those he serves. Let him serve you through the pages of this treatise and let the healing process begin to unfold in your life. Don't allow former disappointments in regards to your wrestling with this condition to deter you from the desired outcome of experiencing a greater quality of life. This book contains a gift of hope and possibility and a link to your longed for future. Whatever has taken place up until now has only made you ready for what you are about to receive. My prayer is that this serves as a pivotal point of a new beginning for you. Let wholeness become your portion. Here's to your health!

Dr. Mark Chironna
Dream Builders Network International
Orlando, Florida

Introduction

If phantom pain and other strange symptoms that seem to have no medical rhyme or reason plague you, keep reading. You may be suffering from a controversial medical condition known as Fibromyalgia. It's hard to diagnose, some medical professionals even claim to believe that it does not exist, but that sufferers are simply making everything up. Thus, those suffering from its "fruit-basket" of symptoms often complains of feeling a little crazy at times.

Muscle pains, aches and pains, headaches, trouble sleeping, memory loss, constant fatigue, intestinal disturbances, emotional highs and lows...do any of these symptoms describe you? Do you think you're going crazy? Does your spouse think you're crazy? Has the doctor written you off as just another hypochondriac? If you're already answering yes to any of these questions, keep reading. This book is for you!

I'll never forget my first patient twenty six years ago. I had just graduated from chiropractic college and had set up practice in a small town in North Carolina. I was so excited. I had just spent six years of college in preparation for this day. I had taken biology, chemistry, anatomy, physiology, neurology, osteology, chiropractic technique, and topped everything off with six hundred hours of x-ray technique. I had taken the grueling National boards, followed by the two-day state board examination. I just know I was God's gift to humanity with healing power in my hands, waiting to be released. But nothing could have prepared me for the person waiting for me behind door number one…

I'll never forget her. Her face will forever by marked indelibly in my memory. I walked into my consultation room on my first day of practice to find her seated amid at least seventeen library books all written about her condition. I realized I was probably in a pickle as I introduced myself, and then quickly excused myself to step out into the hall and ask the Lord to forgive me for my pride. I walked back into the consultation room and began to treat my first patient—who also, as it turns out, introduced me to the strange disease called Fibromyalgia (FMS).

That was over two decades ago. Today we have something called the Internet. I guarantee that if you have been diagnosed with Fibromyalgia, and are also an Internet user, you have undoubtedly already downloaded everything the Internet has to offer on this mysterious disease. There is probably very little I can tell you that you don't already know about FM. But I do know a lot about how the human body works. And I have treated many patients over the years that have suffered with this ailment. I also know the Creator- the God who made heaven and earth, and you too. He provided a way of escape for you from this uncomfortable illness, and I believe He has entrusted me with some keys that may help your discomfort and point the way toward wholeness.

This was never intended to be a deeply scientific book. If you are looking for that sort of book, then this is definitely not for you. But if you are looking for an easy-reading guide to help you navigate rough waters, keep reading. I have tried to make a heavy topic light and easy, and now I advise you to kick your feet up, put on some soft music and read these pages for the hope they contain.

If you have already been diagnosed with FMS and have been told what sort of life you can expect to lead, now that you have it, please keep an open mind. Whenever a thought comes, such as, "Oh, that will never work!" disregard it and keep on reading with childlike faith, the kind that says, "Whatever the diagnosis, today is a new day and there is hope for me!"

And if this is the first book you've read on FMS, it may help for you to realize that you are not alone and that you're not crazy after all! Read on, with the attitude of an explorer, and get ready for the adventure of your life.

-Dr. Timothy Weir, D.C.

Raleigh, North Carolina

Part I: Understanding Fibromyalgia

ONE
"You're not Crazy"

I walked into the consultation room to find a husband and wife sitting there, waiting quietly for me. After I introduced myself, the husband said to me, "You've got to help her, doc! She thinks she's going crazy...and I'm right behind her!"

I wish I could count the multiplied hundreds of times I have heard statements like these over my past 25 years of practice. As I sat down with this couple to being my inquiry into the wife's problems, I jotted down her complaints one by one, then read the list back to her:

- All-over aches
- Headaches
- Pain in the shoulders
- Trouble sleeping

As her story unfolded, tears welled up in her eyes, "I'm not the same person I used to be," she told me. That person, she said, "has long been gone."

Fibromyalgia.

It is so difficult to diagnose, and so controversial in nature, that it's easy to understand why the spouses of its sufferers so often believe their mate is making it all up. And if that's not bad enough, the family medical doctor often supports that view.

Yet, it is my sincere belief that Fibromyalgia is very real, and nothing akin to hypochondria. Because its symptoms seem to come and go and change frequently, the symptoms cannot be fitted into a particular mold. Thus, physicians often ascribe the disease to a condition "all in the mind" of the patient.

A very real enemy
At this point, I like to sit down with my patient and explain just what this debilitating disease is, as I did that day with the couple I have just told you about. I explained to the wife that she suffered from a very real physical ailment, assured both she and her husband that she was definitely not crazy, and told her what I have learned about Fibromyalgia.

"Although it may feel as if you're losing your mind," I assured, "You're in complete control; be confident of that—otherwise you wouldn't be sitting in my office today."

I explained to this patient that she needed to treat this disease as a very real enemy, and come to a complete understanding of the condition so that she and I together could define a battle plan that worked. At that point, I asked her to stop for a moment and consider: "Who is going to win this battle?"

Decide to Win:
What we decide will help us determine our outcomes in life. Therefore, I emphasize the importance of deciding to become whole, in the treatment of my patients. I encourage them to fight to win.

"If you let down your defenses, then this faceless enemy has already won," I said, "So before we go any further, will you commit with me that regardless of how hard the battle ahead proves to be, you will do everything you can to win?"

A tear slid gently down her cheek as this woman shook her head, "yes". At that moment, she and I declared war on Fibromyalgia and she took her first step toward the "winner's circle".

Name that tune:
Remember that old TV show, called *Name That Tune*? If you do, you're probably a Baby Boomer, just like me. But whenever I think about Fibromyalgia, I think about that old TV show because in order to understand the nature of this strange disease, it's vital that we first understand how it got its name.

I am convinced that many doctors affix big, long names to the disease they diagnose, hoping to God their patients never bother to look them up. They hope we'll just take the drugs and not cause any problems. But if we're smart, we'll play detective and find out what we're up against. Things have changed. People are beginning to take control of their bodies and assume more responsibility for their health. As a result, we're asking more questions…and demanding the right answers.

Years ago, people would just go to the doctor and blindly do whatever he or she said to do. The same doctor who birthed them burped them and treated them for life. People kept the same doctor for decades and wouldn't change for anything…but that's not how it's done now. We're a consumer driven society, and that means that today we shop for everything- doctors too.

Dropped Like a Hot Potato!

Those who belong to an HMO have limited choices when it comes to deciding on their personal physician. From a predetermined list of medical professionals, HMO members "choose" their doctor…but if the physician ever ceases to be a member of the HMO, the patient will find that he or she has been dropped like a hot potato.

That happened recently to a patient of mine, who complained that when her insurance program changed, she had to stop being treated by the physician who had been her family doctor for the past thirty years. Because the insurance changed at the company where she was employed, she was forced to find a new doctor, whether or not she wanted one (and she didn't).

Dropped like a hot potato—imagine that! Today, regardless of how great a doctor's "bedside manner" may be, and regardless of his or her credentials, there is so much competition within the medical community that this sort of shifting—from doctor to doctor—takes place frequently. In fact, we've come to think nothing of it. Our parents, and their parents before them, saw the same doctor over and over and over again throughout their lifetimes, unless a geographical move necessitated a change. But this generation changes doctors so frequently that it is now all right to change doctors for reasons other than switching insurance companies.

If your doctor is treating you as if you can't walk and chew gum simultaneously—if he or she is practicing snobbery and refusing to give you credit for being about to understand medical terminology because you're asking for a breakdown of your diagnosis, then it's perfectly reasonable for you to get the yellow pages down from the shelf and let your fingers do the walking through the section titled "Physicians." Find another doctor—one that won't treat you like you are a stupid idiot!

Remember that first patient of mine? She had suffered so much indignity from her doctor, who told her that her Fibromyalgia symptoms weren't real but were all in her mind, that she was relieved to finally discover that the disease was real after all. Thank heaven, she had enough *chutzpah* to keep on pressing for answers, or she would have settled for her family doctor's diagnosis—"It's all in your mind"—instead of mine. I explained about Fibromyalgia and began to treat her for it that day, with outstanding results.

So if you're being treated as if the condition you're suffering from is "all in your mind", maybe it's time to exercise a little consumerism and "shop" for a new physician.

Remember, *knowledge is power.* Use it!

One Word, Three Separate Roots

The Latin roots of the word Fibromyalgia all give insight into the nature of this mysterious disease. Let's explore what the word means by first tearing it apart in order that we may see just what it is you've been fighting all this time.

The first root is the word *fibro*. It's a Latin term from which we have the word, *fiber*. Used in this context, it refers to the fibrous portion of the human muscle tissue. I'm going to digress here for a moment and take you on a mental "walk" through the meat section at your local supermarket. In the section where the rump roasts can be found, think about the last time you shopped for one and found long, white marbleized strands running through the redness of the beef. It's those white strands that compose the fibrous part of the muscle. I don't know how they do it, but these days through the technology known as genetic engineering, cattle are being bred so that less and less fiber will be present in the beef, once it goes to market.

Fact is, we humans have much more fiber present in our muscles, because it's the fiber that gives muscle tissue strength. This fiber acts much like the steel rods placed inside concrete to give it strength.

If we were to examine this fiber in the muscle tissue up close, under a microscope, we would see that it resembles the tightly woven fiber found in the material used to make safety belts in cars.

The second root is the word *myo, or mya,* which is the Latin word for "muscle." It refers to the red, fleshy part of that "rump roast" we went shopping for earlier. It is also composed of multiple fibrous strands. It is red due to the blood that is constantly being pumped through it. We'll talk more about that part later...

The third and final component is the word *algia.* It is the Latin word for "pain." We put together the word "analgesia" from this root word. There is no rhyme or reason to this pain emanating from Fibromyalgia. It is an unusually achy type of pain that can flare up to full-blown sharp pain with absolutely no notice. The first symptom may be something as simple as severe pain in the feet when you first stand up in the morning.

First, The Bad News...
So you've just been to the doctor, and he or she has given you the bad news: "You have Fibromyalgia." Now what?

Don't be alarmed. Your doctor has told you absolutely nothing! You've just been told you have pain in the muscle and its fibers. So what?

I don't know about you, but I'm going to need a little bit more than that. You have pain—that's for sure. Now you'll need to know why you have it, what to do about it, and how long it's going to stay.

And as long as we're talking about roots, notice the word "Fibromyalgia" does not contain the fourth root, *-itis,* on the end. That in itself is good news. It means what you have doesn't contain the Latin word for "flame" - *itis.* What you have will not respond to anti-inflammatories, so don't fall for being advised to taking them by the handful. FM does not respond to those drug therapies.

To beat this enemy, you will need to learn to solve its puzzle, then learn how to put your body back together in the right order. If you don't, you'll have all those puzzle pieces laying about everywhere, appearing to fit together, and yet not. This lack of order will cause imbalances that will leave you with gaping holes where the right pieces ought to go...sort of like a puzzle meant to look like Mona Lisa. If you don't put the pieces together correctly, poor, unfortunate

Mona will be left with a piece of her pinkie finger where her nose should be.

TWO

What it's not!

When searching for a diagnosis, it's as important to know what a disease is not as to know for certain what it is. A case of flu will not respond to treatment for gastritis. If you administer the wrong treatment, you may even wind up with two conditions, the one you started with and the one caused by your reaction to the wrong prescription. Why treat a condition that doesn't even exist?

I like to use this example: If I take my car to the mechanic because there's a terrible clanging going on beneath the hood, it's important to know that it's not the transmission that's falling out, nor the engine that's throwing a rod. How relieved I'll be to learn that the clanging was caused by nothing more serious than a small tree branch that became lodged where it shouldn't have been. No damage! Yet it would have been ludicrous of me to take the car in and order a new engine and a new transmission, when all that was required was the removal of a small foreign object that had been banging around beneath the chassis.

It's the same with FM; it's a disease that can stand on its own, and is not linked with other more serious illness such as Lupus or chronic fatigue syndrome. The proper bloodwork and diagnostic testing will prove that you don't have either of those very serious ailments.

Now, that's the good news about FM: it's not fatal. That's not to say that because of its irritating painful symptoms, you won't feel like dying at times or that at times you might not believe you may even be better off dead!

Hey, snap out of it! Don't give up that easily. As you continue to read, I want to develop something—and that something is called hope.

Yes, there is hope, even for a sufferer of FM…there's even hope for you!

Eenie, Meenie, Minie, Mo!

I can only envision how maddening it must be for the family physician to be listening as his patient drones on about how much pain he or she is in, about how troubled the sleep patterns have been, how tired and irritable and frightened that patient has become…so the doctor begins a rigorous series of tests to determine what the problem may be, when secretly this same doctor wonders if there is any point. *It's probably psychosomatic,* the doctor muses, as he orders another round of lab work.

How, indeed, does a medical professional diagnose such a hard-to-pin down malady as FM? By the "nursery rhyme" method—eenie, meenie, minie, mo? Now, you and I both know that will never work, even if the game is being played out away from the patient, in the privacy of a diagnosis room.

Before I'm accused of coming down too hard on the average physician, let me state that I can imagine how frustrating it must be to be placed in the position of having to diagnose a patient suffering from a panoply of symptoms, all of which refuse to respond to the normal treatment methods. It's not just the patient who wonders if he or she is going crazy. Sometimes the treating physician may feel a little crazy too. After a few months of coming up with "0," he may feel like hiding under his desk when he sees that name of that troublesome patient cropping up on his daily schedule. *Maybe if I just hide under here long enough, he'll go away!* I know how frustrating it is to diagnose FM, because I talk to those doctors and they admit it. In fact, I've heard this statement made by treating physicians more than once: *"Tim, I think I must be going crazy! I just can't figure this one out!"*

Remember, I hear all sides. I listen to the physician confide his frustrations; I listen to the spouse as soon as the patient leaves the room. "How can one person have so many things wrong?" a spouse will often lament. The doctor and patient and spouse, by now, all have at least one thing in common: they're at their wit's end.

There are Guidelines
Because of the numerous cases of FM being diagnosed, the American College of Rheumatologists was prompted to lay down some guidelines. These rules were set down in order to more easily diagnose FM. Yet you may wonder, as I did, *if FM is a muscle-fiber problem and not a joint problem, how come the joint people were given the task of coming up with the diagnostic guidelines?* I think that all the specialties got together in a room and they drew straws...guess who came up with the short straw?

I ask a lot of questions, as you have probably already guessed. But then, it's a necessity in my profession. I've lost count of how many times I asked this one: "Tell me, where does it hurt?" If the patient has FM, the answer is simple: Everywhere!

Three Basic Criteria
The "Joint People" came up with three basic criteria for making the diagnosis of FM.
1. Widespread pain. By definition, this means pain that may be located either on the entire right side of the body (including arms and legs) or pain on the left side of the body (including arms and legs) or the entire lower body—even throughout the entire body. It is very common for a person to experience pain in one area of the body for a while, and then discover that the pain has switched to another locale. Remember, with FM, there is no rhyme or reason!
2. Long-lasting pain. The definition of long lasting in the case of FM is any pain lasting for three or more months. Now, I don't know about you, but I don't like pain. Ten minutes of it is more than enough for me, and to me, ten minutes is "long-lasting." I am someone who considers calling the family doctor anytime I've overdone yard work, so for me to consider being in pain for three or more months makes me want to holler "ouch" at the mere thought of it.
3. The presence of trigger points or tender points. Now, for all you purists, you'll want to know there is a difference between a pressure point and a trigger point and a tender point. Put simply, a tender point is a very tender spot identified by palpation (touch). I hope I didn't lose you on that one.

Imagine coming into my office for a routine examination. As I begin my examination, I push on the trapezius area, and you begin to yell. I just hit a tender point—my definition of it anyway. At this point, you may want to give me your definition: "Doc, if you touch me there again, you're going to pull back a bloody stump!" I just hit a tender point. A trigger point is found when I push on that tender point. The pain may start there but it doesn't stay there. It radiates out from that tender point area and moves elsewhere. Fact is, pain may radiate, and to make the diagnosis of FM, there must be pain radiating from at least eleven of those eighteen points.

See why diagnosing FM is so difficult? Normal testing won't turn it up. It takes a specialist who knows what questions to ask and who can interpret the patient's response to that simple-sounding statement: "just tell me where it hurts."

The Vulcan Death Grip
Remember when the *Klingons* came aboard the USS Enterprise and none of Kirk's men could fight them off? You "Trekkies" will recall that Kirk's strategy was simple: He just ordered Spock to use the fearsome Vulcan Death grip. So, Spock saved the crew by lightly grabbing the trapezius area of the nearest Klingon, dropping him easily to the floor.

Works every time- at least for me, anyway! I don't mean to sound as if I take these eighteen pressure points for granted. The point I'm trying to make is

that these pressure points can cause intense pain—
the kind that can literally rob the body of it's
strength. I have seen strong patients cave in and
slump beneath the lightest palpation of these
pressure points. "Feels like you're using the Vulcan
death grip, Doc!" I've heard more than one of my
FM patients complain. "Lighten up!"

How can I explain that to recoil in terrible pain at
the slightest touch is not a normal response? The
response is not normal, but it's part of what tells us
it's FM we're dealing with. The really frustrating
part is when the caring spouse tries to help by
administering a massage, and they set off terrible
pain by triggering one of these stress points. What
may feel like a normal massage to the spouse may
feel more like the Vulcan death grip to you. How
do you say that? Usually a yelp of "ouch!" will
suffice. It may take you weeks to recover from that
nice massage.

And now a word to spouses: Don't let FM rob you
and your partner of intimacy. Touching is still
okay. Just be gentle. Don't use the kind of pressure
that resembles the Vulcan death grip when a simple
hug and loving touch will do. Learn to work around
FM while you and your spouse maintain intimacy
so that this disease does not rob you of loving each
other and enjoying life.

Three

Somebody Stop the Roller coaster

If there's one thing that distinguishes these pressure points, it's this: They're like a roller coaster. Major ups and downs. Let me paint this scenario for you: You make an appointment at our office and on this day, you are "in the groove." You wake up feeling pretty good, jump out of bed, and notice there's even a spring in your step. When you get to the kitchen you're surprised to discover that your husband has made breakfast for the two of you, complete with a rose in a small vase next to your place setting. He lets you know in no uncertain terms that you are the greatest thing that ever happened to him. He walks you to the car and opens the door for you. As you are driving to the office, you notice how beautiful the day is—the sun shining, birds singing, clouds floating by in the big, blue sky. When you get to the office, your boss lays it on thick, telling you how valued you are as an employee, as he rolls out the red carpet ushering you into your new corner office! "This company would go down the tubes without you!" he gushes as he leads you down the hall to the boardroom for a catered lunch in your honor. Right afterward, you come to my office for an appointment and as I examine you to try to find these tender points, I have a tough time trying to find even one.

According to the guidelines we discussed in the previous chapter, I would hesitate to make a diagnosis of FM after just one such examination. In fact, I'd never make that diagnosis after an exam like that. Four weeks down the road, you're back in my office, screaming about the pain. You wake up feeling like a truck has hit you. Your hubby's in a bad mood, won't even think about making you breakfast, let alone walking you to the car, instead spends an hour ranting about how come you won't pick up his underwear like his momma used to do. The front tire on your car is flat, so you're late for work. Who cares if the birds are singing? It's raining anyway. At work, the boss is waiting for you and starts in about the many reasons why he believes the national debt is your entire fault. In fact, he states it's your fault, too, that his previously stable company has started going down the slippery slope. Why? Because of your lack of sense. Maybe that promotion was premature. Two hours later you crawl into my office and I examine you again, only to discover that of those eighteen tender points, you are suffering from pain shooting out of all seventy-two!

The Roller Coaster
See what I mean?
One day you're up and feeling little or no pain. The next, you're down, with pain shooting everywhere. It's what I call the roller coaster, and you're the one riding it—strapped to the outside of the car as it races along all those sharp ups and downs.

Don't be alarmed, and don't be fooled. When you're up, you feel like you've just ad a miracle and you're finally out of the woods. Then you come down, and begin to explore the forest floor, where you can see firsthand how earthworms live.

I'm very results-oriented. I like to be able to measure outcomes when I examine my patients.

But, when it comes to FM patients, it's hard to measure results from one visit to the next. Because of the roller coaster ride they're on, results may seem to go backward, then forward, then backward again.

On your first visit, you tell me where it hurts. After four weeks of care, I ask you the same question, palpating the tender spots to check for sure. Sure enough, it still makes you scream when I press there. How can I know if you're better, worse or still the same? Believe me…you know and I know. Now instead of hitting the ceiling, you just hit the wall. Progress!

We could list a plethora of symptoms that accompany FMS. Most FMS patients have an extreme sensitivity to smells. You could walk into the perfume counter at Macy's and walk out with a migraine. There are many people that suffer from pain in the TMJ (jaw joint). I have a number of people who start to suffer with night vision problems. The problem is, one day you could be suffering with pain on the right side of your body, then next day no pain, and the following day the pain is on the left side. Trying to figure it out and follow it WILL make you crazy. Just understand that there are a number of symptoms that this disease creates or magnifies. Simply write them down and discuss them with your doctor…if you can keep him from hiding under his desk when you walk in!

Four

I wish I weren't eighteen again!

Remember those guidelines established by the American College or Rheumatology? In that chapter, we learned that there are eighteen possible pressure points that would indicate the presence of FM. In order for a diagnosis of FM to be made, eleven of those eighteen pressure points would need to produce pain on palpation. As I perform my examination, I separate the body into four quadrants: two upper (back and front) and two lower (back and front). In any discussion of these points, I usually begin at the quadrant in the upper back, where some of the most volatile of all the pressure points are located.

The Trapezius Area

Sounds strange, doesn't it? The trapezius area is triangular in shape and made up of the skull down to just below the scapula (shoulder blade). There are two tender points at the base of the skull. These are usually very active points and correlate a lot with sub-occipital (base of the skull) headaches. In case you haven't already discovered, chronic headaches are often among the symptoms of FM. These can range from simple tension type headaches that begin at the base of the skull and stretch up into the head, to full-blown migraines. Neither type is pleasant.

As we follow the map down the trapezius area, we find two points at the very tip edge of the shoulder in the trapezius muscle area. If you live with a lot of stress or have a stressful work environment, these two points become almost impossible to miss. These two points can very quickly become the radiating trigger points if left to themselves.

Once you find these two points, drop down about three to four inches on each side and you will find the next matching pair. These also correlate with extended periods of stress. Before we leave this quadrant, we must travel down the posterior part of the arm, near the elbow, where there are extreme hot spots that may being to affect the use of the arm.

The Frontal Area
The next area to be examined is the front of the body, where the second rib fits into the sternum. This is located just beneath the clavicle, or collarbone. There, you'll find two points you probably never knew existed. You may never have felt pain in this area, but when tested for tenderness, you'll probably fell like going through the roof...at least, if you have FM. If you move from these points to the outside of the neck, at the point about level with the Adam's Apple, you will discover the next set of points.

Then we'll move to the lower body. But before we do, let me give you a scenario: let's say you've had a particularly stressful day. You can really feel those trapezius points flaring up and suddenly your sternum and neck points join the party. As it progresses, the left arm point flares up (to tell you that you used your computer keyboard too much today) and you feel so much pain shooting through you that you wonder if you're having a heart attack. In fact, that's what you tell yourself: "I'm having a heart attack!" So, you drive yourself to the emergency room, where tests are run and EKGs and after four hours, the ER doctor lets you know that you did not have a heart attack. "Must be stress and muscle tension," he observes, as he signs the papers for your release.

What was it that just happened to you? You had a run-in with pressure points that mimic heart problems. Believe me, if what I just described ever happened to me, I'd drive myself to the emergency room so fast that it would make your head spin! And if it happened again, I'd go to the Emergency Room all over again. But if the EKGs kept coming up negative, eventually I would have to face the fact that I was dealing with impostors. And some of the symptoms of FMS are impostors. They appear to be one thing, when in fact they are something else entirely. Just because we find a little numbness in the hands, for instance, does not necessarily mean we're dealing with Carpal Tunnel Syndrome!

THE LOWER FRONT AND LOWER POSTERIOR

Now we move on to the third quadrant. And guess what? Mercifully, we discover that there are no pressure points in that quadrant. Thank God for small favors!

But when we move to the fourth and final quadrant, the lower posterior, we find more than enough ways to make up for that. We begin with the Gluteus muscles. Beginning a the "dimples" just above the buttocks, we work about an inch above and an inch to the side for the first of these pressure points. Now follow the big "ear-shaped" bone around the side, the crest of the ilium, or pelvic bone. When we find this point, we drop down about five inches where the leg fits into the pelvis. Here, we find the trochanter.

To finish our quest to find all eighteen of these pressure points, we go south to the back of the knees. The last two points are found just above the knee joint in the large tendinous area located on the outside part of the knee.

WHY YOU NEED SOME HELP?

Wouldn't it be great if you could examine yourself to find out where it really hurts? Unfortunately, these eighteen pressure points are not so accessible as they may seem. Many of them are located in posterior quadrants and in places where you can't reach. When you try to reach these points, you are actually "using" the muscles that you are trying to test…and that invalidates the testing! Quit trying to do everything yourself! You need some help with this! When dealing with FMS, you'll begin to get stiff and sore and discover that your agility will suffer. Where you could previously reach on your own body, is now out of bounds. This makes it more difficult to check your own muscles.

Best be examined by a professional who knows what to look for and where to look, and best be examined when your muscles are as relaxed as possible so that when those pressure points are touched you don't try to make a fast exit—through the ceiling. I have learned by bad experiences to stand to the side of the patient when checking these points…especially the ones in the back of the knees. I have been kicked one time too many!

Also, be sure that you are checked by someone who knows what they are doing. Just because they have, M.D., D.C., D.O., P.T. or any other degree,

that they are familiar with FMS.   You don't want to
go get someone to check you for these points, and
have to have a book opened up so that they can
locate them!   My God, can you imagine that.
Believe me, I have heard it all!   Just ask the
receptionist on the phone when you are making the
appointment if the doctor is familiar with FMS.

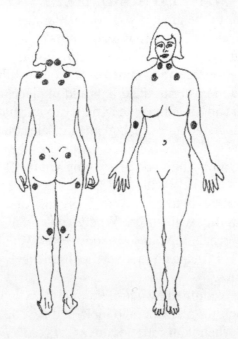

As you can tell, I took the art course on the back of
the cartoon books. Here are the 18 FMS points!

FIVE

What to Do When the Fog Rolls In!

There is another strange condition that's commonly associated with FMS patients, and it is called "brain fog." I just don't like that term. I prefer to call it short-term memory loss. If you are right now reading this book and wondering why you ever bought it…perhaps you're experiencing it! It is a very frustrating, confusing, and scary part of the overall condition called FMS.

Imagine walking up to your best friend of twenty years and as you prepare to introduce her to someone else who just walked up, your mind suddenly goes blank! You cannot remember her name, no matter how far back you reach for something that will jog it into focus. You couldn't remember her name even if you were threatened with bamboo slivers shoved under your fingernails. It's as if someone had taken an eraser and erased her name permanently from the chalkboard of your memory. You tarry for a moment, buying time, until the awkwardness of the moment passes. Then, twenty minutes later, it hits you. BRENDA! That's it! So what? She's long gone and you're still feeling pretty stupid. The harder you try to remember in those situations, the deeper the hole gets! Here is a key for you…when this happens just relax and start to laugh. Make this moment as light as you can. When you do this, it allows you to get to where you want to get faster. But if you sit there and try to fight it, you will frustrate yourself beyond measure. Short-term memory loss. It can hit you at the grocery store, the mall, in class, at the office, and especially at home. Your husband may tell you that you are going to have dinner tonight with the Rogers so be ready no later than six P.M. SHARP! When he gets home, you're sitting in the den with your bathrobe on, watching the news. You completely forgot. Where'd that information go about dinner at the Rogers. It went in one ear and out the other and got lost in the fog. It probably is in the washing machine with the missing pairs of socks.

I can always tell FMS patients at the mall. They are out in the parking lot with their car lock "clickers" up in the air, pointing it waiting for the horn to beep. They forget their computer passwords or the ATM passwords. Yikes. That could make you want to beat your head up against the wall. DON'T DO THAT!

IT'S SO SCARY....
I was in consultation in my office with a very successful trial attorney, who began to cry as she told me how scary this short-term memory loss associated with FMS had become. "Can you imagine how it feels to be standing in front of a judge and jury and forget where I am and what I'm doing?" she lamented. I told her I couldn't imagine. "It's horrible!" Many times people will tell me that they will be up in front of a gathering of people doing a presentation, and in the middle forget where they are at in their presentation. They don't know what they have already said, or what needs to come next.

Short-term memory loss. It hits at the worst times…and when you're in the midst of a stressful work situation, the instances intensify. The boss tells you to do something and you forget…adding more stress.

If you are experiencing short-term memory loss…brain fog…the best thing you can do for yourself is to relax. No, you don't have Alzheimer's or some other pathology that is escalating in severity and terminal in nature. Yours is simply a symptom of FMS, and it comes and goes, much like that rollercoaster of pain we discussed in an earlier chapter. You are merely experiencing short-term lapses in your ability to recall facts and events. The more uptight you get about these lapses, the worse the condition will become until it finally subsides…until the next episode.

Don't hide your experience from your family and trusted loved ones. It is vital that you communicate what you are going through and reach out for their support. Educate them as to what you are experiencing and get them involved in finding ways to help you stay on track. I highly recommend that you have them read this book. Remember, I did not write this book for professionals…I wrote it for regular people. I made it fun and easy to understand for this very reason. I want those people around you to understand what you are facing. I also recommend that you somehow get this to people around you who may be wondering why you do and act the way that you do. This may be a pastor, teacher, boss…but above everyone else, your spouse and family need to hear this. If they still don't understand, get them on a plane and fly to Raleigh and meet with me in my office. I'll make sure they don't leave until they know what is going on.

Now, practically, I recommend to my FMS patients that they carry a small pad of paper with them containing a header that goes something like this:

Things to remember today….

Then start to list them, one by one. Write down little things one would normally remember easily—such as where you parked your car at the mall or airport. When you park at the airport, write your parking space number or area on the parking ticket, and carry that with you. Please don't do that and then leave it in the car. Put it in your wallet so that you can retrieve it quickly. Believe it or not, a lapse of memory over a little thing like that can cause a huge amount of stress until the memory returns! And how about other little things like your computer password or ATM pin? Write those things down and carry them with you so you'll avoid stress later in the event that the fog rolls in…..

SIX

I Can't Take Another Late Night Infomercial!
Imagine being so dead-tired that you lay down to
sleep and then find that you can't! Sleep, that is.
Your eyes are heavy and you ache everywhere.
You're bone weary and yet can't drift off to sleep.
Your body just won't give in and let you rest. This
condition is known as non-restorative sleep, and it's
another common symptom of FMS patients. I
would consider it an almost cardinal symptom, and
a huge key to helping with getting free of FMS.

In the FMS patients I have seen throughout my
years of practice, I have seen three manifestations
of this condition called non-restorative sleep. These
are:
1. IMMEDIATE SLEEP. The minute your head
hits the pillow, you're out cold. You don't move a
muscle. But an hour and a half to two hours later,
it's as if your eyelids rolled up like shades at the
window. You're wide-awake and staring at the
ceiling and unable to go back to sleep. At this point
you will toss and turn, moan and groan, and do
anything but sleep for the remainder of the night.
Finally you doze off about five A.M....but the
alarm goes off at 6:00! A new day has started, but
you never were able to finish the previous one!
2. CAN'T SLEEP. Your head hits the
pillow...and nothing happens. You try to close
your eyes but they won't stay shut. You stay up
watching every infomercial and rehashed talk show
on late night TV and can recite most of these scripts
by heart. You feel like your skin is crawling and
you finally doze off...at about four-thirty. Again,
the alarm breaks your blissful reverie at five-thirty

and by then, you're so tired, you just want to crawl into some dark cave and finish sleeping.

3. LIGHT SLEEP. Your head hits the pillow and you fall asleep at 9:00 P.M., and you sleep all night until 8:00 A.M. You sleep all night long but awake feeling as if a truck has hit you. You feel worse in the morning than when you went to bed and that's even if you slept 12 hours! If you think FMS is confusing to your family, this is one of the big kickers! How could someone sleep 12 hours, and get up for an hour and have to take another nap? No wonder they think you are crazy!!

FMS patients never make it through all four of the normal phases of sleep, to that stage known as deep sleep when the body is most relaxed. It is that fourth phase, also known as the REM (Rapid Eye Movement) state, that people dream. As the eyes move rapidly back and forth beneath the closed eyelids, people are actually "watching" their dreams unfold on the movie screen of their eyelids.

CAN WE TALK?
Remember that frustrated spouse of my first patient? I mentioned at the beginning of this book how, the minute my patient left the room, he looked at me and started to confide all his frustrations, pleading, "Can we talk?" It is hard for family members to understand how someone who looks good on the outside, can feel so bad on the inside.

He wanted to know how anyone could suffer from so many strange aches and pains. He also wanted to know how somebody who went to bed routinely at 8 P.M. could wind up feeling at eight in the morning as if she had no sleep! "She needs a nap as soon as she brushes her teeth!" he complained to me that day. "How can that be, Doc?"

It is at this point that I always have to explain the strange manifestations of non-restorative sleep.

Consider this scenario:

You drive home from work and park the car in the garage, go inside, do a few chores, have some supper, watch a little TV, spend a couple of hours on the Internet, then go to bed and sleep until 7 A.M. when the alarm goes off. You get up, shower, shave, and dress for work, then have breakfast. You kiss your honey good-bye and walk out to the car, get in, and prepare to drive to work. But as you stare at the dash, you realize there's no gas left in the car because the night before when you drove into the garage, you forgot to turn off the ignition. The car engine was running all night and used up all the gas. The car's energy source was depleted and so now you'll have to take a cab.

All that energy depleted. FMS does the same thing when we can't get the sleep we need to function properly. When most of us drift off to sleep, we relax and enter a deep state of rest. FMS patients don't do that. All night long, they're using muscles that they don't need to be using. There's that constant state of tension. Problem is, all that tension is using up there "gas"—energy. They awake feeling drained and as tired as when they went to bed the night before.

OUR FACTORY MAINTENANCE PROGRAM
One of the most wonderful things about our Creator is that he mad provision for us in so many magnificent ways. Sleep is one of those provisions. Consider that deep REM sleep state as God's "Factory Maintenance Program." Nightly, as we

drift off to sleep, bound for the REM state, God is waiting to meet us there and recharge our batteries, give us a quick tune-up, and prepare us for another day's output. Any factory worker will tell you the importance of shutting down for the night so that more work can be accomplished during the day. Our body needs a break too. In order to get it, we need sleep so our organs and muscles and intricate network of veins and arteries can shut down And operate at less than full capacity.

When most of us go to sleep, we hit that REM state, where the most rest and relaxation occur, and where the most restoration takes place in order to prepare us with the energy we will need during the next day. The REM state is also where essential routing maintenance occurs such as basic healing and repairs that go on while we are sleeping. FMS patients are different. They rarely hit the REM state. Instead, they spend the night tossing and turning, using muscles they don't need to be using, creating that constant state of tension that results in more pain. Problem is, all that tension is using up valuable energy that could be used for other, more important things. It uses up our gas so that when more energy is needed to perform life's essential tasks, the FMS patient is too weary to accomplish them.

That built-in restoration system doesn't work so well for the FMS patient. See why getting into that deep sleep state is such a priority? By now you've probably guessed that while I'm a proponent of good health, I recommend natural means versus drug therapy when at all possible. Even if you need sleep badly, why take a pill to put you to sleep when it will take until two in the afternoon to shake off the drug's after-effects? So the question is this:

What can you take safely that will not harm the body, but actually help its natural healing process to occur?

HOW TO GET A GOOD NIGHT'S SLEEP
Here's my prescription for a good night's sleep: First of all, it's important to make certain that you're in a room that's conducive to sleep. A dark room is best. I love going to those really nice hotels where the curtains are four inches thick. When you draw them during the day, the room goes totally dark and you can sleep till dark if you like. It's dark enough that you won't know what time of day it is.

Don't forget, when you are sleeping, or in the process of falling asleep, the brain is still taking in information. You are hearing and recording everything that's going on around you, and your brain is logging all that data into its memory banks. If you leave the TV on with the news blaring, you'll be recording all the details about hose three killings, ten car accidents, five bank robberies, seven rapes, and fourteen hijackings. Your brain is left to process all that garbage. May I suggest that instead of sleeping while the TV blares, turn if off and turn on a tape or CD of some nice, relaxing music, or perhaps an inspirational selection or motivational speaker. These choices are better for you and will help you to relax while uplifting and restoring your soul.

I am also going to recommend that you take a nice walk right before you go to bed. We live in a society that is extremely introverted. What I mean is, we sit in front of computer screens for hours on end, or we sit at a desk and focus our attention on a phone and memo pads. Doing that for hour after hour, your mind gets narrower in its focus, it becomes introverted. Then when you get home, you sit down to eat, and then you sit in front of a TV watching it for hours, and then you go to bed. You have completely introverted. Then when you lay down to sleep, you are still in an introverted state, so your mind stays there. Your mind continues to replay your day. You remember every detail of every transaction that took place. You go back through all the phone calls, all the emails and every other thing that you did. The problem is…your computer is not turning off! How do you "reboot"? You get extroverted. Extroverted? Yes, you get your mind to focus out further than inside your mind. How do you do that? I highly recommend that you go on a nice long walk. Go out and walk in the great expanse of creation and just look. Don't walk with your eyes looking down at the ground! Look at the trees and clouds, look at the dogs playing and the stars. It is amazing how your mind will expand when you realize just how small you are in the whole of life! You also begin to understand that we are all connected. You begin to have cognitions of where you have been and where you are going. I believe that unless we extrovert, we become so introverted, that we forget that we are just a small part of a bigger thing! It becomes all about me….instead of me being a part of a whole! Get out in the sweet evening air and let that oxygen fill your lungs, and that oxygen will get to your brain, and allow you to sleep a deep sleep.

In another chapter, we'll discuss nutritional supplements that will help you sleep soundly all night through!

SEVEN

DID THIS MAN SIN, OR WAS IT HIS PARENTS?

There is a Bible story in which Jesus heals a blind man, then answers the question of one standing nearby—"Who did sin, this man or his father before him?" Did his own sin, or the sins of his parents or grandparents cause the man's blindness? In other words, was the man's blindness hereditary in nature? And did generation sin cause the man to be born blind?

I can't count the number of times, in talking with FMS patients, I am asked the question, "What did I ever do to bring about this disease?"

Did you do anything to bring it upon yourself? The answer is usually no! The more I have learned about the human mind, the more I do understand that it is possible that you have done things to yourself and others, and are holding that against yourself. Can doing that cause disease? Sure. It gets to a point where you "punish yourself" for the things that you have done. You do things to others, and then don't tell anyone about it. So, we end up with two things....first, the thing that you did wrong, and secondly, not telling anyone about it. As crazy as this sounds, we feel like we have done so much, that we could never be forgiven. The fact is, some of this may go back even to your childhood. I think sometimes that we brush things under the rug so many times, that we don't deal with our "stuff". I think it's time that we face what we have done and deal with it. This is called confrontation. The ability to confront things in your life. A good place to start with this is just by writing down your "trespasses". Those things that you have done to others or yourself. It is amazing how sharing this, brings things to the surface and removes many heavy burdens. We often feel that if people knew the "real" us, the person who did some things in the past, that they wouldn't love us, or want to be with us! Maybe not! But guess what? You're getting to the point where you don't want to be with you either…so correct it! Confront those hidden areas in your life. That may be stealing a piece of candy from the corner store when you were a kid, or having sex with someone other than your spouse. If this stuff is not dealt with, eventually you get to the point where you believe that the only relief is to "leave this body." That is sad! The fact is, there is no "sin" so big or bad that it deserves you having to die!

The problem then becomes the second part of this thing… "not telling anyone about your trespass." Listen, I have been in church long enough to see what happens when you tell people secret things. Within days, it has gone to the board of elders, deacons, their wives and the church secretary, finally you get the church newsletter, and it is on the front page! That then makes it impossible to unload these hidden areas! Did you know that there are actual Internet sites that people can go to and share some of their hidden sins? As crazy as that sounds, it literally allows people to unload a lot of burdens. Once you have written down your "transgressions," if nothing else, send them anonymously to me. You will be amazed at how freed up you will feel.

IS THIS HEREDITARY?

There is much speculation about whether this disease is hereditary or not. Many times there is a grandmother who suffers, and her daughter, and finally you! Does that prove it is hereditary? No. What I have noticed is that we tend to "mimic" our parents. We take on their traditions and habits. We tend to take on their exercise and eating habits. So, if your mother never ate a lot of protein, but ate a lot of breads and pastas, you tend to eat those same things.

Then where did it come from? Let me share some of my observations gained from treating thousands of patients afflicted with FMS. First of all, we find FMS mainly in women, and I believe that there are a few reasons for that. One may be related to the amount of serotonin present in the nervous systems of women compared to men. Serotonin is the chemical produced by the body to help it deal with pain. If something happens to upset the delicate serotonin ratio, the body will have less defense against pain and the patient will become more sensitive to the pain reflex.

Also from my observation and study, we see FMS occurring more frequently among women who have had some type of female surgery—hysterectomy, tubal ligation, breast surgery, abortion and yes, even the birth process itself. All these traumas to the body seem to affect the ever-present hormonal flow to the body. The upset of the hormonal balance is enough to throw the person in to a tailspin. Don't forget that it's the hormones that are the keys necessary to turn on and off all other systems of the body. These hormones affect the nervous system, digestive system, respiratory system, pulmonary system, and endocrine system.

The human body is a delicately balanced masterpiece that can be upset by outside intrusion.

OXYGEN-The Life That is in the Blood!
It's blood that makes our tissues appear red beneath the skin. The life of the body is in the blood, because blood is the "highway" that carries vital oxygen to all parts of the body. Without the proper oxygen, the tissues of the body will begin to wither and waste away. The brain literally will starve without oxygen. It is possible that there may be some type of oxygen deprivation that leads to the kind of starvation of the muscle tissues correlating with FMS. It is also probable that such oxygen deprivation is one of the causes of FMS. This may come about in any number of ways. It is possible that there has been some type of chemical or toxic substance that has been breathed in for an extended period, or there could be chronic asthma. Do you remember having had asthma? I remember as a child, we would go camping in Northern Wisconsin in the summer. In those campgrounds, every night, the "bug man" would come…you know with the toxic chemical fog to kill mosquitoes. The problem is, we would get on our bikes and ride through that fog. Kinda stupid now, but back then, it was awesome. That crazy little stunt over a period of weeks is enough to cause oxygen deprivation problems.

TRAUMA
Consider some type of traumatic onset—surgery, or the long and difficult birth of a child. A tremendous amount of force is absorbed in the body by such traumatic events. I think these events are about the same as being rear-ended by a car. Such

accidents release a great deal of force, and our body absorbs the shock although it appears that afterward there are not visible injuries. After all, there are no broken bones or bruises or laceration to the skin. But how about the unseen injuries to those connective tissues that keep us held together? How about the unseen shockwaves to the tiny fibers—those muscles and tendons—that have been stretched or torn and now are sending out signals of pain?

FMS patient often complain of such pain, and when they describe it to me, it reminds me of the kind of pulling and stretching that's required in the making of taffy candy. First the taffy mixture is warmed, the pulled slowly until it forms thin strands. Then it is pushed back together and warmed some more, and pulled again. The more the taffy is pulled and stretched, the easier it is to pull apart the next time, and the softer it becomes. Of course, its softness and pliability is part of the charm of taffy. The taffy would become brittle in the process if heat is not added. In the stretching process, it would literally be torn to pieces in a cold condition.

But our muscles aren't taffy. Consider what happens to muscle tissue if it's pulled quickly without ever warming up first. Like that taffy, the tissue would be torn to bits. Now imagine what happens to these soft tissue structures at the point of sudden impact in a rear-end collision. One minute you're driving and totally relaxed behind the wheel. The next, out of nowhere, a car speeds up from behind and its impact throws you forward and into the dashboard area and then slams your head back onto the headrest. Without warning and no "warm-up," those relaxed muscles are pulled like cold taffy to the point of breaking as your head snaps forward, and then backward. The problem with ligamentous tissue injuries is that when healing occurs it heals with fibrous scar tissue.

NO ONE CAUSE
It is my opinion that not one but several of these events, in combination, cause FMS. Any form of stress that the body encounters for a prolonged period of time is a form of energy that the body must deal with. The body will inevitably follow the path of least resistance. That's the law of nature. That stress will not go down into the bone material because it's too impenetrable. So the next areas to be attacked with will be the muscles and soft tissue areas—even the skin. That's why skin eruptions become so evident in people experiencing chronic stress.

Why not do a quick inventory on yourself? Are any of these elements present in your case?
❑ Accidents in the past? Car, falls, slips?
❑ Reproductive surgeries
❑ Oxygen utilization problems? History of Asthma or Emphysema?
❑ Chronic, prolonged stress? Bad marriage, bad job?

It is important to know where you've been so that you can begin to chart your future! There yet may be situations you will need to correct so that you can move forward into better health and away from the things identified as stressors. You can learn to walk out from under all that stress you've been placing on your body. How important is that career if the stress it causes makes you constantly feel like you're dying? Let me answer for you; it's not worth it because life is too precious for you to let it pass you by…

I have been lambasted by religious people when I tell my patients… "if you are in a bad marriage… get out!" Listen, the only person that you have to be accountable to is you! "Oh, God hates divorce". I'm sure He does, but I cannot believe that He loves it when His children suffer in a relationship that is harmful, hurtful and painful. Abuse isn't just getting hit on your body! It also is abuse when you are verbally attacked day after day. It is abusive when someone tells you that you are a lazy, good for nothing wife." This is one of those areas where you need to count the costs and figure out if this relationship is worth being sick over! I've heard of being "love sick"…but this ain't it!

I am also amazed at the amount of people who are doing things for a career that they don't want to be doing. Maybe their parents made them do it, or they got stuck doing something on their way to the "real thing" that they wanted to do. Let me make it simple…if you get up in the morning, and you aren't excited about going to the office, or company or the shop to do what you love….CHANGE!! It is never too late! I had a nurse who always wanted to be a chiropractor, but felt like she had spent too much already to be a nurse, and was now "older." I told her that it would take her 4 years to get her D.C. degree. She said, "In 4 years, I'm going to be 44 years old!" I said, "True, but let me ask you this….if you **don't** go to chiropractic college, how old are you going to be in 4 years?" She said that she was going to be 44. True! Whether you venture out and do what you want or not….you're still going to be the same age. Guess what? She got out of the boat and walked on water! She is

now a practicing chiropractor. Enough said?   Sure.
Get out of the boat!!

THE ONLY THING YOU CAN CURE IS A HAM!

Okay, I was a bit hesitant to bring this up, and that's
why I waited until about halfway through this book.
Who like to be the bearer of bad news? And who
like to receive it, for that matter? But if we're
going to continue being open and honest with one
another, I must tell you openly and honestly that
there is no known cure for FMS.

   You need to know that there is no magic potion
or pill to swallow that will affect a quick fix. Being
completely rid of this horrendous disease is not
going to happen, short of a miracle.

   But here's where hope comes in: You can learn
to manage this condition and by that, I mean, with
proper guidance, you can live a relatively normal
lifestyle.   You can learn to get off many of the
drugs that have been covering up your symptoms
and get on with your life.

   Are you ready to start on the road back to
health?   Don't get me wrong, this is not an easy
trip, like a cruise to the Caribbean!   This is a rough
road with a lot of potholes in the road, but the fact
is, it is worth every step.   This is not a trip for the
weak hearted…but the trip is worth it!

   I am constantly amazed at how many times I get
things from people that claim to cure
anything…almost grow hair on a cue ball. Sorry, it
just doesn't work that way. There is no magic pill
or drink…there are a bunch of things that if done
together…they will help you get back to
Healthville.

So rather than look at this through magic rose colored glasses, we are going to look at this with multiplex glasses. There are a number of areas we need to look at, nutrition, nervous, psychological…all of them parts of an extremely multifaceted disease. Don't freak out on me now. Let's just sit around the kitchen table and plan out a strategy for you to get well. OK? OK! Do me a favor. Be willing to put away all your preconceived beliefs and be willing to experience some new things. Be willing to say that some things may sound so simple ….almost too simple to work, and be willing to do them!

EIGHT

THE JOURNEY BEGINS WITH THE VERY FIRST STEP

Someone once stated, "The longest journey begins with a single step." So it is with FMS. Our Journey toward managing it and making life worth living again also begins with a single step. But the first step we make in any direction is also the hardest. The fact that you bought this book and have read this far means you have already made a decision to improve your life. There-you see? You've taken the very first step. You made a decision, and that's like laying down the gauntlet and letting the "powers that be" surrounding you know you're serious about making some changes. In making the decision to change your lifestyle and start managing FMS instead of being controlled by it, you're in effect saying, "I am not quitting, stopping, laying down, giving up, shutting off, or cooling down. I'm in this for the long haul and I am going to WIN!"

I can already hear some of you saying, "But you don't understand! I've been fighting this thing for ten years without success. I'm tired and afraid that I'm stuck where I am and so should just make the best of things." Some of you have gotten to the point where you are almost already dead…but you just haven't had the grace to lay down!

Not so! That old adage that states, "Today is the first day of the rest of your life," can be applied from here on out it you'll just make the commitment to make a few changes. Decide now how it's going to be, should you live another twenty to thirty years. What will it be—a lifestyle filled with pain, misery, and defeat? Or a lifestyle filled with power-packed, overcoming victory? The choice is yours. Is that hard for you to believe? Believe me…that is the truth. The fact is, the point you are at right now is a decision that you made and chose to believe years ago!   Want to change your future? Then you must change some decisions that you are making today!!

THE GREATEST BATTLE
 My dear friend, Dr. Mark Chironna frequently states that the greatest battle any of us will ever fight is the one between our ears! Forget being attacked by evil forces or even the devil himself. Most of us are our own worst enemies, and over and over again we defeat ourselves in the battleground of our minds long before we ever enter into battle with another opponent.

Today is a day of destiny and if we're going to win, we must decide to be on the winning team. That means we must stop attacking ourselves with doubt and reasons why nothing is ever going to change. We must stop analyzing everything and start making changes based on the simple belief that we will have an excellent outcome!

As with most enemies, you're going to have to play to win. You must be ruthless with yourself and refuse to keep believing you're defeated. Separate yourself from your FMS and now that you are not the disease. Over the years, I have watched patients take on the identity of diseases and get lost in that. "I am a diabetic." No you are not. You are a human being that suffers from a condition called diabetes. You are a wonderful person who happens to be plagued with FMS. If you cannot separate yourself from the disease, then in order to get rid of the disease is to get rid of yourself!! Wow. Quite a difference. If you can separate yourself from the FMS, then and only then can you be ruthless with the disease and attack IT as a separate entity instead of attacking yourself. You didn't cause this and you can control it. We'll see how to bring relief in coming chapters.

EXAMINE SOME OLD ISSUES
Some may find relief from pain in also examining some old emotional issues. Jesus said we must love our neighbors as we love ourselves, but sometimes people have a hard time here because they may find they love their neighbors more than themselves. But that doesn't work. We feel guilty because we feel it is wrong to love ourselves. Truth is, if you don't love yourself, it is impossible to love your neighbor. Take an emotional inventory as you begin this process toward better health habits and examine where you are. When you look into the mirror, do you love the person you see reflected there? Some of you right now are having some cognitions as to why you may have had some of the relationship problems that you have been having.

Some of us are even mad at God because of how we came out of the oven. We judge ourselves as too fat or too skinny or too tall or too short, too much hair or not enough, too brainy or too…well…not brainy enough! We wish that we looked like somebody else…but God made you to be just the person you are. Learn to be content with being you.

Learn to celebrate who you are. You have a destiny. Accept that. You are an incredibly powerful being. Sometimes we allow people to talk us out of how powerful we are. "You shouldn't

think of yourself more highly than you are!" How many times have you heard that? Who told you that? I'll tell you…some jerk. If you have been told that you'll never "amount to anything," or anything else negative, you need to have a mental enema. You need to flush out all the crap that has built up over the years, and replace all of those little sayings with sayings that build you up and allow you to be the powerful being you were created to be! Look at all the things that you were told over the years. Start with your parents. Did they build you up or tear you down? Tear down…dump that stuff. How about teachers? I'm told that Albert Einsteins teacher told him that he would never amount to anything. Aren't you glad that he didn't listen to her? How about preachers? There is a certain amount of control involved with someone who wants to keep you a lowly worm…unable to think for yourself. Listen, it is time to step out from under the "thumb" of every controlling person in your life…and swell up to be the powerful, creative being that God made you.
Quit worrying about going to hell if you do…my God, you're already there. It is time to break out!

I encourage people taking responsibility for their own lives. Quit blaming God and the devil. Find out what you are doing that is not right, and set it right. You will be amazed at the power that you get when you realize that you are in the control seat. Don't like where you are? Just change it! EASY!

FEEL GOOD?   GREAT! ENJOY IT!!
The minute that I mention exercise to my patients,
their whole countenance changes and they begin to
grimace. It is if I mentioned a dirty word instead of
one that could result in better overall health! The
problem is, the minute I mention the word *exercise,*
memory kicks in and the patient begins to recall all
those times they put themselves through untold
torture in the name of fitness only to fall back,
exhausted and defeated with little or no real lasting
change. I used to offer a workshop to the public on
FMS, and often the poor spouse would be along for
the ride. They try to be supportive, but honestly,
they are getting a little tired. Usually when I got to
the point of talking about exercise, I could see the
spouses elbow jab into the ribs of the FMS patient,
and as they leaned over, I could hear them say, "I
told you, that's all you need to do is exercise." It is
amazing to see that people hear what they want to
hear. True, exercise is important, but listen to me,
the very part that you are trying to exercise is
diseased. When you try to exercise, it causes those
muscles to overreact.

When you try to exercise, the brain pulls out all
of those old tapes of the last time you exercised, and
the time before that, and I hear comments like, "I'd
rather be stuffed in a box and dropped over Niagara
Falls!"

One reason exercise fails is that we fail to use it
properly. We tend to either over-exercise…or not
exercise at all.

This is a big problem with ALL FMS patients!
It's not just you. Consider this scenario: You're
having a fabulous week. Tuesday through

Thursday, you're riding high. The FMS is barely noticeable and by Friday morning, you announce to your hubby, "Honey, I feel so good I think I'll vacuum the carpets." You pull out the vacuum and start in on the living room. As you work, you notice some spots that you decide you can't live with. So, it's down on your knees with the cleaning fluid to take them out. Then you decide to jaunt off to Ace Hardware store to rent a steam cleaner so you can really do the job right! You arrive home with the super-duper, deluxe model steam cleaner and 300 gallons of carpet shampoo and you decide that while you've got it rented, you'll do the whole house.

Then while you're at it, you decide the car needs it too, so after you've finished the house, you steam clean all the carpets in the care. Then you hand-wash and wax it, and hand-clean the windows, inside and out.

Speaking of windows, you want to get everything right, so you start in on each of the windows throughout the house, cleaning each one by hand. And as you're finishing up the exterior windows, you notice the exterior of the house could use some of that elbow grease, so you spontaneously decide to power-wash the house. Back to the hardware store to rent one, along with a twenty foot extension ladder.

While up on the ladder you looked down at the yard and notice it could use a good manicure, so you come down, cut the grass, and till up the backyard to make it ready to plant annuals. Then you plant them!

Get the picture?

When Honey comes home at 6 P.M., he has been fantasizing about the awesome night on the town you guys can have, because finally....you feel good. He announces he's surprising you with a night out on the town and you just collapse, unable to move your lips and just to say NO! Finally, you form the words, "Just get me to bed! I need to be in the horizontal position!" You're beat to a pulp, and of course you can't sleep. You also can't move a muscle. Who's fault is it! Yours! You over did it, and its going to take at least a week for you to recuperate. The problem is, now you have added another problem...a break in the relationship communication. No wonder there is a problem!

   If the last time you exercised you tried to do it all, all at once, until you were as worn out as the above scenario, that's probably the tape that will play each time some well-meaning health professional mentions the word exercise.

   Am I right? Yes.

It Doesn't Have to Be That Way!
FMS patients miss it if they kept the philosophy, "I'm having a good day, so I'm going to cram it full! After all, I don't know when I'll have another one!" That's the wrong philosophy because it is based on past failures. It leads to overdoing followed by long recuperative periods. Find your limits, then stay within them and you'll build yourself up through regular exercises. For the adage, "no pain...no gain!" does not apply in the case of FMS! I would like to give you permission to do something...NOTHING!!! If you are having a good day, enjoy it with the thought in mind...there are plenty more of these ahead! Let me give you permission to enjoy the day. I give you permission to go to a movie. Find a chick flick, and go! Yes, just you! WHAT? During the

day? Sure! While the kids are in school…go to a movie. Not shopping, not working…not cleaning….movie!! Guilt? Over what? Enjoying yourself? Oh brother, you have more mental enemas to take!!

Here is another thing I want you to consider. How much does your family spend on going out to eat? Let's be honest. For a family of 4 to eat at a good restaurant, you are going to drop at least $50-60.00. Now, if you are like most families, you eat out at least 2-3 times per week. If you can sit your family down, and ask them to eat at home for 2 of those meals per month, you can save that money, and then hire someone to come in and clean your house once a month. Once a month, they can do the major cleaning. If you save 4 meals a month, you could have your house cleaned 2 times a month. Holy Cow, that would be enormous! Can you imagine having someone clean your house every other week? I just save your body a major cause of FMS Flare-up! You don't have to be a movie star to have your house cleaned…just creative financing!

Exercise also does not necessarily mean joining a gym and keeping up expensive membership fees. People lose it when they begin to conjure up visions of themselves in yards of Spandex, working out for hours on end until the sweat pours off. One of my patients proudly told me that he had just spend hundreds of dollars on a stair-stepper machine. I cringed, then asked, "Do you have stairs at home?" When he said yes, I said, "Why didn't you just use them?" People think that they have to spend money on a membership or equipment…but you don't have to!

Forget expensive memberships and elaborate gym equipment. Just find something rigorous that you like to do, and do it! Take the dog for a walk around the neighborhood. But the trick is, do it consistently, until it is a routine. I counsel my FMS patients to do a little exercise on a regular basis instead of overdoing it a bunch of it at once, and then regretting it for days afterward!

Try purchasing some five-pound weights and incorporating them into a basic exercise program. But don't do a hundred reps. Start out with five reps and NO MORE! It may sound silly and worthless, but starting out easy will help you stay at it until you build a little more resilience. Go to Target, and look in their sporting goods section. You can buy some pretty cool stuff there to get started. Remember, you are not installing a gym in the house. You are just going to get some weight to put under the bed! Don't forget that they are there! Remember…Five (5, cinco, nickel, one, two, three, four, FIVE, funf, cing) reps! No more! Is that a deal? Promise me!

When I began my practice 25 years ago, I was naïve. I prescribed all sorts of exercises and when my patients said that they would do them…I believed them. (I believed in Santa Clause until 2 years ago!) That was until one day I prescribed exercises to a particular lady, and watched her go to her car. She looked the sheet over, and flung it over her back, into the back seat of her car. I caught on and changed how we do things. Today, we have a rehab department at the office, and we sit with out patients and watch them exercise. It's important to know how to exercise properly, since exercise is all about strengthening the soft tissues. If not done correctly, exercise will strengthen the wrong areas while not helping the areas that need help. At that point, it would be better to not exercise than to do it wrong!

You may need some support in order to stay with it. Why not team up with a friend? Get an I-pod and listen to some supportive programs. Go to our website and download some of my Power Living Radio Podcasts. Get some nice music and listen to it. Listen to music that speaks to the soul. There are some great jazz musicians or pop. I am very choosy to what I listen to. I'm not going to listen to songs that talk about losing my job, cheating on my wife, and not paying the bills. Holy Toledo! Get songs that will build you up...not pull you down. This is a great time spend time with your spouse. Talk as you go. You want to be able to talk. If you are too out of breath to talk...slow down! This is a great time to build relationships. The time and distance will pass quickly as you build stamina and better fitness. But make sure that you wear good walking shoes. Please don't walk in flip-flops!!! If I see you out walking with them, I'm going to grab them off of your feet and beat you over the head. Now, I'm not getting paid for this, but I have always used New Balance shoes. Their walking shoes are incredible. They provide a great foundation to the feet.

Start out with success in mind and that's what will surely result. Find something you like to do, and do it . Walk the dog, park the car further away from the stores at the mall. Take the stairs instead of the elevator. All of these things will create opportunities for exercise. See? You didn't need that gym membership after all!

Are We On The Same Page?

Dear Friend, I could spend hours and pages talking about what people believe FMS is, and how they got it. The fact is…the jury is still out. We do know that it is real and it is a bona fide disease. It even has it's own fancy ICD-9 code for diseases.

I have heard it all! I have heard the theory that all FMS patients were sexually abused as children…that is why they are dealing with this disease. That is preposterous. Did some FMS patients get sexually abused as children? Absolutely. There is no doubt. Did ALL of them? No! Do all children who are sexually abused get FMS? NO! Again, there are hundreds of different traumas in ones life. We need to quit lumping people all into one group. This is one of the most exasperating diseases encountered.

The interesting thing about this disease is that what works for one person, makes another person worse. If I were to tell you that there is ONE way, and no other, that would be a lie. There is no one thing that works. It is a combination of things that sift out into the exact thing that works for you.

All right? Lets get to the answer!

PART II: Let's do something about it!

NINE

Testing: One, Two, Three...Testing.

You're in pain, and you've tried everything...without success. I can empathize. I've talked to hundreds of FMS patients who had tried everything else by the time they came to me. Most all of them admitted that this was their first experience with alternative care. And because of the excellent results in the management of their FMS symptoms, I am convinced more today than ever that there's a need for this often-overlooked therapy.

If you think about it, it's easy to understand why FMS would respond to something like chiropractic care. After all, the pain that accompanies this disease affects virtually all the body's soft tissues— areas of the body that ware controlled by the "Master Communication System," the nerves located along the spinal column. The nervous system, although "plugged in" to the spine, is vital for the proper function of not just muscle and tendon tissue, but all of our organs and virtually every other system of the body. All of them get their "orders" from that master communication system.

Someone once said to me, "I think it's preposterous for you to claim that a chiropractor can do anything to help FMS! That's a muscle-fiber problem and you deal with nerves. I just can't buy that!"

I felt like saying, "I'm not selling anything for you to buy!!" But I didn't say anything. I have found that usually people who are argumentative, are usually so pig headed, that trying to talk to them about anything is like talking to the a brick. However, statements like this do not deter me from believing that chiropractic care is a key to improved health for FMS patients. It merely demonstrates the attitude that many people have about my field of healthcare. It clearly displays the reasoning of those who try to "compartmentalize" the body, when all parts of the body are actually under orders from the nervous system—my area of specialty.

PUTTING TO REST THOSE UNFOUNDED FEARS

So let's discuss some of those unfounded fears that people seem to have about the chiropractic field. I see the blood drain from some people's faces at the mere mention of the word chiropractic. "If you go to a chiropractor you could end up in a wheelchair! I know…because I heard it from my cousins' brothers' mail-mans' sister."

Believe me, I've heard it all, and statements like these reveal unfounded fears that have no basis in reality. Many of those who most fear chiropractic therapy are the ones who would not even flinch if their family doctor told them that they were going to try an experimental surgery for memory loss that involved taking out the brain and injecting it with steroids, and then re-implanting it into the skull. They would not refuse those seventeen experimental drug prescriptions for a disease, 16 of which have serious side-effects, including death. Yet, they balk at an approach to healthcare that helps the body to heal itself…simply performed by the gentle manipulation of the vertebra in place. Go figure.

Today chiropractic therapy has become so refined and safe that it's **results**, not **side-effects** that you can expect to receive. Many of the low-force techniques now in use are especially safe. I use a combination of a couple of techniques. One of which is the Activator Methods technique. This uses a small adjusting instrument that gently taps the spine and the accompanying muscles that effectively moves the vertebra into place. This has been used for years, and is incredible. Just recently I added the Pro-Adjuster to my repertoire of methods. This technology is based on data from NASA that uses an instrument to check the integrity of the joints. If the joints are "stuck", it will cause a change in the computer. Both of these techniques are more aimed at making changes in the nervous system than moving bones. So, you may go, and wonder when the chiropractor is actually going to do something. The fact is, if you can change the nervous system, the bones will move!

Do yourself a favor and quit believing the prophets of doom who warned you about chiropractic therapy. Realize that many of these people also talk bad about nutrition, exercise, acupuncture, massage and anything else that is not stamped with their own approval stamp. Many of them make judgments from hearsay and not from their own experience. Then, look around your city and find a chiropractor that uses one of these techniques and get going!

PUTTING TOGETHER ALL THE PIECES

The great thing about modern medicine is that there are so many state-of-the-art tests available to help physicians in their diagnoses. Take, for example, rheumatoid arthritis. The doctor can run blood tests and find things in the blood work alone that will detect RA. It is the same thing with Lupus and Lyme disease. Then x-rays and an MRI will correlate that diagnosis with more confirming clues. Cardiac problems can be diagnosed with all sorts of tests including EKGs, blood work, and spirometry, so that within minutes, the doctors know what they are dealing with.

Not so with FMS. There are no conclusive tests, no MRI findings, and no orthopedic and neurological exams that will definitely diagnose this condition. It is a disease of what I call, "last man standing". You must rule out all of the other diseases that mimic FMS, like Lupus, Lyme, and RA, and then check the 3 criteria from the American College of Rheumatology, and if they fit, bingo, you have found your missing puzzle piece.

An interesting thing began to show up during my first couple of years treating FMS. Of course, being a chiropractor, I rely on x-rays in many of my diagnostic findings. In about 99% of the cases of FMS, I find a correlation of loss of the neck curve and a thinning of the C5/6 disc space. That curve is vital to the health of the entire nervous system, and when it is absent the neck becomes weakened.

Inside the spinal column, a protective sheath called the Dura Mater covers the spinal cord. It is attached to the top of the spine and the bottom of the spine. When the neck curve is missing, there is a stretching of the Dura Mater. In my opinion, it is this stretching that causes the painful flare-ups associated with FMS. A chiropractor will find these problem areas after proper testing, when a medical doctor might miss it because he or she is looking elsewhere to solve the puzzle. Standard testing won't net results with this tricky disease….SORRY!

Can you see why your family doctor is so frustrated by this disease? There are no absolutes. Sometimes it just takes someone willing to step out on a limb and let you know what you are suffering from! Again, if your doctor doesn't even acknowledge the presence of FMS…go find someone who does. No need sitting in a room with someone who doesn't believe you.

TEN

Health Food: No Longer Just for the "NUTS."
We first began to hear the term "Health Foods" in
the sixties, and we Boomers who happened to be
around then probably began to associate the term
with the tie-dye T-shirts, bell-bottom jeans, and
long-haired peaceniks who seemed to be the chief
proponents of the "Health Food" craze. Health
foods—wild hickory nuts, pinecones, trail mix---
that's stuff for nuts! I remember going into a
health food store back then, and smelling the
incense and all of the natural foods. I was waited
on by a lady with dreadlocks, and more underarm
hair than King Kong. Honestly, I thought I was
caught in a bad episode of the Twilight Zone.
      Back then, anyone into health foods was
considered to be "way out" by the rest of society.
We called nuts anyone who ate health foods, while
we hit the fast-food lanes and ordered up our
burgers and fries and charbroiled side-items.
      Today, however, health foods are no longer for
"nuts." It's not only acceptable, but fashionable to
be watching what you eat. If you visit a health-
food store today, you won't find many hippie-types
in tie-dyed-T-shirts and bell-bottoms jeans.
Instead, you're more likely to find professional men
and women in upscale business attire, loading up on
healthful items like humus, soy products and tofu.
Health-food stores are thriving as they sell
everything from vitamins and natural dietary
supplements to organically grown vegetables and
beefsteak.
      Scary? Perhaps not! Today's popularity of
health-food stores is in keeping with how a greater

portion of the population is beginning to take responsibility for their own health and well-being. What we eat matters, and as a society, it appears that we have finally come to realize that a daily diet of drive-through burgers and fries does not make Johnny healthy, wealthy and wise. It makes Johnny sicker than a dog!

PROCESSING ALL OF THAT POISON

We humans are indeed, "Fearfully and wonderfully made," as the psalmist David wrote. (See Psalm 139:14) but the way we were made never took into account that our bodies would be forced to process pounds and pounds of poison annually. Poison? That's right; all of those additives to the food products we find on the grocery store shelves, all those preservative, are nothing more than poison to the human body. It was, after all, designed to process vegetables and fruits, meats and nuts found in nature. Only in the last century did we begin to process foods with chemical additives that we concocted in laboratory test tubes.

Right now, your body is working hard to process that sandwich that you ate for lunch today. It's removing what nutrients and vitamins were contained in it, while scrubbing away the poisons and removing them through your liver and kidneys. Whatever fuel is left is being broken down and distributed to the parts of the body in need of energy. If your sandwich contained protein, perhaps that protein will wind up going to help rebuild a portion of the retina of the eye. The fat has probably already been taken in, and used to give you that burst of energy you felt right after you ate.

Now, if you topped things off by eating a toaster pastry, a can of cola drink, and an ooey, gooey chocolate bar, let me give you the bad news! Your body can take in stuff like that for just so long before it begins to give out. The empty calories in those items won't help rebuild your body a bit. It's a little like trying to rebuild a computer's hard-drive using parts you find in garbage cans. It doesn't work to use all kinds of trash to build diodes and transistors. And sure enough, it won't work using garbage to maintain your body.

I was appalled when I first went to my son's school, and saw what they had in the cafeteria for the kids to eat. For kids who had breakfast, they had pastries and orange juice…pure sugar. For lunch the kids got either a sandwich or a "nacho plate" and then they could have either cookies or cake, washed down with some type of kool-aid drink…again…pure sugar. There was a point where kids could go to a vending machine and get soda drinks and chips. Did you know that there are 16 teaspoons of sugar in a 12 ounce can of the "yellow" soda drinks…plus caffeine. It is no wonder our kids can't sit still in the classrooms. What do we do? Change their diet? No…we give them some type of mind-altering drugs designed to make their behavior more tolerable! Yikes. I'm concerned about our future. Not happy? Take a drug. Too happy? Take a drug. Depressed? Take a drug. Can't concentrate? Take a drug. Someone has to stand up and scream… "STOP THE CRAZINESS!"

GOOD EATING EQUALS GOOD HEALTH!
It's not too late to start eating right! Good eating, equals good health, in my opinion. I recommend a low-carbohydrate diet. As you increase good proteins in your diet and decrease carbohydrates, you will find your muscle tissue will benefit almost immediately because proteins are the building blocks of muscle tissue.

Eat lots of good vegetables. May I also suggest that you immediately begin to cut out some of the garbage foods that you have been eating. Stop the sugars and refined carbs. It is amazing the effect that sugar has on the nervous system….let alone the pancreas and endocrine system. It is just not worth eating those little frosted cakes for lunch everyday. Now listen, I will indulge in a little something every once and a while, but a lot of us have gotten to where it is daily. Your body just can't take that!

THE LESSER OF TWO EVILS
Now listen, I am really not a friend of sugar. I believe that it has caused much of our degenerative disease in this country. But much worse to me are the artificial sweeteners on the market. These things are deadly. They will cause symptoms from migraines, muscle aches and seizures. There are only a couple of things that every FMS patient has to do in my office….this is one of the biggies! Get off all artificial sweeteners. There are two of them that I believe are less problematic than the others, one is Sweet-N-Low, the other is Stevia. Between these two, the Stevia is by far the best. There are much less side effects with that than any others! I had an MD friend whose daughter was in a wheelchair with what they thought was MS, but no

diagnostic tests to back that up. Off the cuff, I asked her if she drank any diet drinks. YES! She drank a 2 litre bottle OR MORE everyday. We took her off of those drinks and within 2 weeks, she was up walking normally! It is that bad. Please do me a favor, pour that mess out, throw out the packets, and just drink water.

Of course, I also deal with people who want to be natural in their diet, so they substitute honey for the sugar. Can I tell you something? Your body doesn't know the difference between honey and white sugar. It is all sugar. So, don't fall for that one. If you need a sweetener, either use a small amount of sugar or stevia. OK? OK!

I highly recommend starting out your new lifestyle by adding just one serving of vegetables at lunch and dinner. This may be as simple as adding a salad. Be careful of the dressing here though! If you have IBS, you want to be careful of eating lettuce….especially iceberg. The cells that make up the lettuce tend to be rather hard on the intestines. Use Romaine lettuce with some tomatoes and cucumber. I like to just get some olive oil, which is great for your cardiovascular system, with some nice Balsamic Vinegar. Remember…NO CROUTONS! I also like to add some grilled chicken to that salad to really balance it out. Eat a lot of chicken, fish and lean red meats. If you are a vegetarian, then you may want to reconsider being one! Evidently that is not working too well for you! You're body is craving protein, and you will never get enough eating what you are eating. For years Dr. Atkins was ridiculed for his diet, but the fact is, many people are healthier for it.

You must be extremely careful with caffeine products. These include cola drinks, coffee, tea, and chocolate. This not only interferes with sleep, but it also affects muscle tone. Adding a chemical that increases these two problems just doesn't make sense. It's just not good for you. Again, don't freak out. Certainly a cup or two of coffee a day isn't going to hurt anybody….it's the people with 2 or 3 POTS a day that I worry about!

But if you're already thinking, Dr. Weir, I just can't give up my chocolate bar in the afternoon! I recommend that you stop right now and make an important decision. Is that thing that you are craving worth feeling depressed and uptight, stiff and sore, and unable to sleep tonight? Why not do this…ask your family! I don't think it is.

MAN SHALL NOT LIVE BY BREAD AT ALL!

There are two basic problems with bread.

Now you will really want to throw the refrigerator at me for this one. For those of you suffering with FMS, wheat can cause a severe allergic response. You hate me, I know. Listen, I grew up in Wisconsin, and if we didn't have some kind of bread with every meal, there must have been an atomic attack. My grandma Johnson baked fresh bread for us every single week. Not just bread… homemade rolls, cinnamon rolls, and any other type of roll that you could think of. I mean, this is the kind of bread that would make you want to slap your momma! She made the most incredible bakery items. I remember getting up early in the morning on that day, and she had already started her mixture. I can imagine it right now, and I can still smell the yeast. She would cover the dough, and stick it over the heating vent for it to rise. Do you know what it is like to give up something that you think you cannot live without….sure.

There are two problems with bread. Let's deal with them one at a time. First of all is the wheat. We find so many times with FMS an allergy to wheat and wheat gluten. Let me give you a couple of the symptoms that accompany this wheat allergy. Headaches, dark circles under the eyes, chronic coughs, blood sugar problems, stomachaches, gas, fatigue, muscle aches, depression and the list goes on. You find that kids with this allergy eat it, and then act out of control. They whine and cry. The intolerance to gluten, is an inherited disorder that comes form a sensitivity to the part of gluten called gliadin. This little guy acts as an antigen, and it will combine with antibodies that lead to an immune complex in the intestines. There is an entire cycle that happens, and much of it has to do with the production of PGE2 (Prostoglandin E2), which leads to the end product of inflammation in the tissues. This inflammation is the root cause behind joint pain, muscle pain and if you have kept up with the cardiac information….heart problems.

So what does this wheat thing include….or should I say exclude? Bread, pasta, pastries, donuts, flour and everything made from flour. It doesn't stop there. I want to give you a list of some hidden sources of gluten. Flavored coffees, some candies (like strawberry Twizzlers) and even some types of vinegars. The key is to really learn how to read those food labels.

Now Dr. Weir, I was "with you" all this far, but now this has gone just too far! I REFUSE TO GIVE UP MY BREAD! Oh really. How selfish does one have to be? You refuse to give up your bread, so you lay in bed for days whining about how bad you feel…making your family suffer through your suffering. That my friends, is the epitomy of selfishness. You better get over this love of bread and get into the love of life!

What's left to eat?

What do I eat? I highly recommend that you eat mainly lower fat meats, vegetables and fruits.   Plan your meals with lots of vegetables. Let me give you a sample menu for one day.

BREAKFAST
2-3 eggs (if you scramble these, put in some onion and green pepper with some cut up left over steak)
OR
A low sugar, low glycemic indexed protein shake

MID MORNING SNACK
Either a piece of fruit
OR
A low sugar, low glycemic indexed protein shake

LUNCH
6 oz of cut lean meat
Side salad with some olive oil and Balsamic Vinegar with some cukes and tomaters (southern)!!!
Cut up veggies

MID AFTERNOON SNACK
Fresh veggies with some ranch dressing
Cheese cubes
OR
A low sugar, low glycemic indexed protein shake

DINNER
8 oz of lean cut meat
Stir-fried veggies
Side salad with olive oil and Balsamic vinegar

Now that isn't that bad is it? Try this for 30 days, and just see how you feel. I know that you will feel more energy and less pain. Then try a test of some wheat. You will be amazed at the way your body reacts to this. Believe me, it will be just like you have ingested some poison....well actually you have. Give yourself 30 days.

Don't Forget the FAT!
It is incredible to see what people eat. They might just as well eat slab of cardboard. They are so afraid of fat. Remember, it is not the fat that kills you, it is the combination of fat and carbs that does you in. I was raised in Wisconsin, so butter was a big thing for us. The fact is, butter is an incredible source of Omega 3! It is really good for you! If you compare it to margarine, which is one chemical reaction away from being plastic....it is awesome. Plus it tastes so good. Now...this doesn't mean an entire stick on a piece of toast...but a couple of patties sure wouldn't hurt!

The second problem with the bread is the yeast. We have noticed with FMS, a tremendous problem with yeast overgrowth in the body. This will manifest in many ways, but one of the worst side effects is fatigue. You have to be extra careful about any type of fermented foods that are high in yeast content. For those of you who like an "occasional beer," this has a double-edged problem…high sugar and high yeast. You better to stick with just water to drink. There are a couple of good products on the market to help you get rid of the yeast build up in your body. Go to a good health food store, and tell them that you are looking for something to combat yeast. I highly recommend Pau-D'Arco tea. This is a tea that you can drink, but it doesn't taste that good. Drink it anyways. This is a problem that you need to deal ruthlessly with, and it may take doing some things that you don't like doing. Tough!

ELEVEN
Herbs, Vitamins, Homeopathy…Confusion

If you want to really get confused, go to your nearest health-food store and take a look at all the stuff they have for sale. You can take something for anything, and most health-food stores have it…even pills to help reverse hair loss. But what should FMS patients take, and how much? Just trying to figure out the directions on the labels of the various pills and potions offered there may cause you to run out of the store, screaming in frustration, "Where's the nearest donut shop? I need a dozen and a cup of coffee!"

When you are dealing with a condition as complicated as FMS, with so many various symptoms, you must be careful what you take into your body as a form of therapy. Just because a product includes the term "natural" on its label, doesn't necessarily mean it's good for you, or that you should take it! What about its side effects? And how will those side effects further complicate your FMS symptoms? Extended use of vitamin A, for example, can have toxic effects on the body.

I've peeked inside some people's medicine cabinets and 300 bottles of pills have fallen out--- pills for everything. Beware of getting in too tight with that neighbor who sells XYZ vitamins on the side and swears he's got just what you need to cure your every ill. It takes years to learn how different vitamins work together, and I'm particularly leery of Chinese herbs. They can cause serious side-effects if not used correctly.

ESTABLISH A FOUNDATION

Taken correctly, vitamin supplements can provide a foundation that will lead to good health. Before you do anything else, I recommend that you add a good multivitamin formula to your daily diet regimen. That multivitamin should contain the maximum daily requirements of each of the following:
B Vitamins
Beta Carotene
Calcium
Magnesium
Zinc
Potassium

In addition, I recommend that you also use a food formula to aid in oxygenation. At the top of the list of possible products is vitamin E. The Proanthocyanidins found in red wine grapes are also important in this formulation. You will find that with regular anti-oxidants, blood flow to muscles will increase, as will blood flow to the brain.

THE NUMBER ONE PRODUCT I USE FOR TREATING FIBROMYAGLIA....RELAX!

I'm talking about the formula I came up with using magnesium, vitamin c, vitamin d, potassium and MSM. There is not choice if you come our clinic! If you have FMS...you have to get on this. This does just that much! I recently had a man try this who works with people all day. He has to make sure that he is well rested. The first day I gave him a sample, and he begged me the next day for more. He got an incredible night of rest. You will love it too.

**ONE A DAY VITAMIN PILL?   YOU HAVE
GOT TO BE KIDDING!**
Please don't be duped into thinking that you can
take all you need of this in one little pill.   That just
doesn't make sense. You need a lot for your
foundations….one pill worth is not going to do it.
Find a product that combines a bunch of good stuff
in packets.   Buy some of those little "Glad Snack
bags" and fill them up with your daily dose. You
may have to get a shelf that is set aside for just your
pills. Find the ones that work best for you and add
them to your own little formula.

Natural Help For All Those Symptoms!

If you have been fighting something as painful as FMS for months on end with little or no results, you should be relieved to learn that there are some things that you can do for yourself to bring improvement---things that will help restore you to good health with few, if any side-effects. The following are my recommendations of natural means to combat FMS. These vitamin and herbal supplements can be found in most health-food stores and are relatively inexpensive, while the results they bring are beyond price.

I have studied homeopathic medicines and nutrition, and have personally observed the positive effect of these treatments.

Let's begin with learning how to beat the blues…and you don't have to be an FMS sufferer to have a case of those from time to time!

DEPRESSION

We all get low feelings from time to time. A little dip in the mood from time to time is nothing to worry about. But when our feelings dip and stay there, we call it "a case of the blues." Psychologists, however, call it depression and physicians counter it with prescriptions for mood-elevating drugs like Elavil and Prozac.

I can tell you from experience with some of my patients that the blues will definitely accompany FMS at times. I recall a recent consultation with a beautiful twenty-five-year-old patient who was forced to reduce her work schedule to twenty hours a week because of the debilitating migraines associated with FMS. Her fiancé said she had become very depressed over this decision and confided, "We just need some hope."

This thing called depression must be dealt with for the enemy it is---swiftly and ruthlessly. It is dangerous to allow it to linger, when there are things that you can do to eliminate it. I'm not talking about the occasional "down" days; I'm talking about the "down" days that come to stay.

FIRST, inventory your surroundings and remove all the negatives you possible can remove—including friends. Don't let those around you drag you down. Life is too short. Surround yourself with people who will build you up, edify you, and make you feel as if you're going to make it.

Next, reduce your intake of negative newspaper, TV and radio broadcasts. Focus on positive uplifting things.

THE HAPPINESS FORMULA. This is a little regimine that I put together for people with mild to moderate depression. Are you ready?
In the morning…start with 500 mg of vitamin C and 400 IU of vitamin E. At night, take 100 mg of B1. Do this for 2 weeks. At the end of two weeks, at lunch, add another 500 mg of vitamin C and 400 IU of vitamin E and then at night add another 100 mg of B1. Do this for 2-3 weeks, and then add one more dose of 500 mg of vitamin C and one more vitamin B1 at LUNCH! You will be amazed at how you will feel much clearer and leveled out. If this doesn't do it for you…then
FINALLY, consider adding one or more of these herbal treatment for increased well-being:
❑ St. John's Wort—hypericum is the actual name of this herb, nicknamed after John the Baptist. It's

been used for centuries to treat mood swings and help with sleep disorders. It is not a cure for clinical depression, but simply a mild mood elevator. It gives an overall feeling of well-being, and does not come with side effects generally found with prescription medications commonly used to fight depression. St. John's Wort can help mid to moderate forms of depression. I recommend one 300 mg capsule three times a day for a total of 900 mgs. If that dosage seems to mild to net results, try two capsules in the morning, one at lunch, and one at dinner. St. John's Wort sometimes causes mild phototoxicity—skin sensitivity when exposed to sunlight. If you are fair-skinned, you may want to avoid exposure to sunlight. If you do go out into the sun, be careful to wear some type of sunscreen. St. John's Wort is not to be taken with any other form of antidepressant. It has some characteristics of monoamine oxidase inhibitors, so do not take St. John's Wort if you are already taking an MAO inhibitor!

GINKGO BILOBA
This great antioxidant will help increase blood flow and also help with headaches, short-term memory loss, and depression. I recommend starting slowly with 60 mg per day, building up to 180mg per day. You will probably note excellent results if you suffer from a harmless condition known as tinnitus (ringing in the ears) and may also find that this herbal treatment also helps if you have numbness in the limbs, dizziness, or asthma. It is a great herb to help a lot of problems.

PYCNOGENOLS
These antioxidants are mead from either grape
seeds or pine nuts and help increase the blood flow
as well as oxygen that is used by the body.

FISH OILS
I highly recommend taking these as we have
previously discussed. If you are feeling depressed,
than get on a daily dose of these. I would
recommend 8-10 pills per day. Is that a lot? Not
really. But you will notice that it will cause you to
enjoy life more. If you are going to take these,
spend the extra money and get a good brand from a
health food store. Here is a little clue: If you burp
fish after taking them, freeze them first. It will
make all the difference in the world. These are
vital for children to take also. I have noticed that
kids with ADHD respond very well to these.

B1. This little guy is an amazing help in the time of
need. Here is the protocol: start with 100 mg per
day. See how you do. If it helps…then add in
another 100 mg in the evening. This is especially
important if you are one of what I call "night
worriers". These are people who lay their heads
down, and immediately their brain begins to go
through senerios of things that have absolutely
nothing to do with anything of any kind whatsoever.
I mean someone may have said to them that day, is
that a little mole on your face? Dang…by the time
2 a.m. comes, in their mind they have diagnosed
melanoma on themselves….they have gone through
surgery, chemo, radiation and plastic surgery. Of
course, that is not enough! Who is going to take
care of the children? Is their husband going to
want to remarry? Who is going to sing at their

funeral? Should the casket be open casket or closed? Maybe they should be cremated! But….the problem with that….when Jesus comes back….will He be able to find her if she is just a jar of ashes!!!! The next morning she gets up, and that zit has come to a head! Imagine this…wasting an entire night, not able to sleep over a ZIT!!!   You need some B1.   Go to a good healthfood store and get a nice size tablet.

WHEAT IS AN ENEMY!
So many FMS patients are allergic to wheat, and one of the biggest side effects is a feeling of depression.   You will see a little later that this little bugger causes a host of problems.   Do yourself a favor and stay away from it for 3 weeks and see for yourself if it doesn't make a difference.

CAN WE TALK ABOUT IT?
 Finally, get in with someone that you can talk to about this. As you can tell, I am not too hot on Psychiatrists. They don't listen…they write scrips for dangerous drugs. Find a counselor that will spend time hearing you out. The fact is, there may be things in your past, that you have been trying to cover up, or trying to go around and not deal with. Now is the time to deal.   We are so afraid that if people knew the real us, they wouldn't like us any more.   That is a lie. Find someone confidentially that you can confide in, and share your past…to get you to your future.

Again, find someone who is not the church gossip.
Sorry to say, that might not be your pastor. Can't
tell you how many times someone has gone to their
pastor, and within hours it is back to that person. It
has gone through the "prayer chain". Sure! Or
worse…it is preached from the pulpit the next
Sunday! Wow.
You may have to get out of your comfort zone to
find some help here.

SHORT TERM MEMORY LOSS

There's help for "brain fog" too! First try limiting your intake of TV. The brain needs a workout just as much as any other part of the body. Instead of an evening in front of the tube, try reading a book. Make reading a habit by setting the goal of reading a book a month., or perhaps even a book a week. Pick out something you like and read. Start the day with a few selections from a motivational book. Read things that will increase life inside you…not pull you down. Do a crossword puzzle while listening to some great classical music—perhaps Mozart or Vivaldi. You can enrich your mind as you relax and because you are keeping it engaged, your mind will have less opportunity for the fog to roll in.

Also, weed your diet of things like Honeybuns and candy. Your brain takes in enough garbage without feeding it garage too! Choose foods that nourish the brain, foods rich in protein and vitamins. An all-carbohydrate diet will actually contribute to memory loss, while eating more proteins will increase your memory capabilities.

As with depression, Ginkgo Biloba really helps reduce brain fog because this herb contains the active ingredient, ginkogoflavonglycosides. This helps keep damage from free radicals to a minimum, while increasing mental agility. I recommend 40-60 mg of this. Results should be measurable within four to six months of usage. You will notice that you are thinking more clearly and having less trouble with short-term memory loss.

I also recommend the addition of the following herbs:
Gingseng
Black Cohosh
Bee Pollen

CHOLINE—used three times a day, this will help increase acetylcholine, the message-transporter of the brain

NIACIN—This is vitamin B3, but you must be careful taking it. It greatly increases blood flow to the brain, and you may even be sensitive to niacin. Many people experience a "niacin flush," which includes a hot feeling all over for about 15 minutes. This is a harmless reaction, but can scare the mess out of you if you don't know it. Start out with a very small amount. I recommend starting out with 100 mg per day, and build up over several weeks. This is also great for helping to reduce high blood pressure.

PYROXODINE-B6, taken at 50 mg per day for about a month, will help improve your memory. It is also wonderful for symptoms of numbness associated with Carpal Tunnel Syndrome. After the initial month, take the B6 in quantities listed with your multivitamin.

VITAMIN C—This is a wonderful antioxidant and a natural anti-inflammatory. It also improves circulation. I recommend the addition of 3,000 mg per day. It may cause stomach and/or intestinal disturbances like diarrhea. If that happens, simple cut back on the amount, but keep taking the vitamin C. If you bruise easily, you should especially add more to your diet. The deficiency of this important vitamin will cause blood vessels to become fragile and so bruising is more frequent.

OXYGEN
Now listen, I think oxygen therapy would be of great benefit to most FMS patients. It stands to reason…more oxygen…more brain power. So how do you increase the oxygen to the brain? Here is an easy exercise…ready? Take in a deep breath and hold that for 10 seconds. Do this every 30 minutes.

Now here is another no-brainer. If you need oxygen, quit doing things that decrease the amount of oxygen in the body……SMOKING! Ok, it was ok to try a couple of times when you were a teenager, but if you are still doing it at 35…you need to be taken out back to the woodshed. I am amazed by people who are so taken back when the doctor tells them that they have emphysema or lung cancer and they are smokers. Holy Cow Batman…what does it take for people to smarten up? What is even worse, then they try to sue the tobacco company for giving them cancer. Wow. First of all, it just doesn't make logical sense to take hot smoke into your lungs, day after day, year after year. Secondly, how many times do you have to be

warned?   THIS IS YOUR LAST WARNING!!
STOP!

COENZYME Q10-
This like other substances is found in the body.
The problem is…in you….there may not be enough.
Here is another clue! If you take statin drugs to
lower your cholesterol….then you definitely are
deficient, because they strip the body of Coenzyme
Q10. It will affect brain function, but it also affects
the muscles. This one thing alone may make you
feel like you have Fibromyalgia. I recommend that
you take 100-120 mg per day. Stop on the way
home and get some of this stuff. Again, just find a
good health food store near you and buy some. Not
the cheapest, but it doesn't have to be the most
expensive either.

PHOSPHATIDYLSERINE- This is incredibly
important for brain function. It is involved with the
neurotransmitters that are responsible for quick and
accurate thinking. It is important to note, that as we
grow older, our store house of PS is depleted, and
we begin to lose our ability to think like we used to.
We sit and stare at the walls trying to remember the
name of someone we have known all of our lives.
Take 180-200 mg of this per day, and see how it
rolls. As with most things, give it a good 6 months
to build back up in the body.

B12- I love B12. It is great for energy and also
maintaining the integrity of the nervous system. It
helps promote the myelin sheath around the nerves.
This is like the plastic covering around wires. If
that covering gets messed up, so does the message
that is going down that wire.   There are different

ways to take it, I like the sublingual or liquid B12.
500 mcg per day.

SLEEP DISTURBANCES
Probably one of the most frustrating of all the
problems related to FMS are sleep disturbances. I
have discovered that if we can work together to
solve that one, many of the other problem
symptoms will be greatly helped. There are a
number of possible causes to these sleep
disturbances, including possible drug interactions.
List the drugs that you are currently taking, and then
look them up in the *Physician's Desk Reference* to
make sure that you are not experiencing counter-
reactions. If the answer is yes, then ask your doctor
if there are alternate medications.

   Prescription drugs, even those recommended to
enhance sleep, will leave a person so groggy the
morning after that it can hardly be considered
healthy. The idea of a giant green moth landing on
my face kinda gives me the heebee jeebees. That
makes me a little claustrophobic. My thinking is
like this…if you have to take drugs to put you to
sleep, then wake you up, and then another to
energize you, you are not human anymore…you are
a walking pharmacy!!! Let's try to figure out ways
to naturally get you some good sleep.

   Try this…an hour before you go to bed, go out
and take a nice walk. Again, this will help get you
from being so introverted, and it will help you relax.
When you get home, have a nice hot cup of
chamomile tea. Now, if you have allergy problems
to ragweed, etc, stay away from the chamomile tea!

   I'm also recommending that you don't eat too
late in the evening. When you realize that your
body is a food processing plant, your "factory" has

to stay open until that food is processed. Your last meal should be eaten no later than 7 P.M. I know this is a bit redundant, but stay away from the caffeine this late at night. Don't drink a double fricko hottie latte, and expect to go right to sleep. That is suicide. If my wife drinks a cola at dinner…no sleepy that night. So be careful little mouth what you drink!

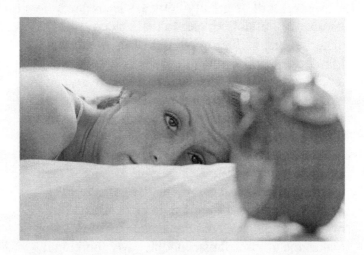

What do you need the most?
RELAX FORMULA. This great tasting beverage helps you relax, and helps the computer shut down at night. Many people note that it helps their joints too! Order this from our website today.

SLEEP APNEA

Before we go any further, we need to address a very serious issue. This is Sleep Apnea. It literally means "no breathing" while you sleep. With this condition, there is a problem with breathing so that sufferers do not get a good night's sleep because they are continually awakened by their breathing patterns. They literally stop breathing several times during the night. People are very weird about this condition. It is amazing. They will deny it to the death that they have this. Most people deny snoring. "No, I do not snore." Well of course you can't hear it…YOU ARE SLEEPING. Those affected with Sleep Apnea may be sleeping, but they are not resting. If your family says that you sound like a Craftsman Chainsaw…then you need help. I fought this for years. My family said I sounded terrible. You could literally hear my snoring upstairs behind closed doors. One summer, we went to Chicago and stayed at the beautiful Embassy Suites downtown. My kids were in the "living area," and at midnight, they made me get up and get my own room because they couldn't sleep. It was MIDNIGHT!! There were no rooms…I had to go 3 blocks away to another hotel. I was embarrassed, but it got me off my butt to get it checked. It kept getting worse. I would stop at traffic lights and doze off. What did I do? I went to a sleep lab and had a sleep study done. You spend the night in a room that looks just like a hotel, except that there are wires and things all over the place. So, they hooked me up, and within minutes, I was sleeping. What I thought was minutes, was actually hours, when they woke me up. It was 2 A.M., and they had enough data supporting the fact that I had Sleep Apnea, so they wanted to finish the study with me hooked up to a CPAP machine. (Continuous Positive Airway Pressure) This machine goes over your nose, and actually forces air into your nose and that keeps your airway open. I woke up at 5:30 totally refreshed. I went home and awaited the results. In 2 days, we got them. I had Sleep Apnea. I would be sleeping, but then arouse myself from sleep by snoring or stopping breathing….24 times per hour!! It was no wonder that I fell asleep at my desk. I was sleeping…but I wasn't sleeping!!! Since wearing the CPAP machine, I am a different person. I am rested and once again…ALIVE! If you know someone who snores or if you do yourself…go get a sleep study done. Ask your doctor, because not only are you not getting sleep, but you are putting yourself at risk. Why? The 4 biggest side effects of Sleep Apnea are these: 1. Strokes 2. Heart attacks 3. Diabetes 4. Stupidity…seriously! Literally millions of brain cells are killed off every night from a lack of oxygen to the brain.

Obesity will also affect your sleep. Your throat is being choked by the excess weight. I notice that my wife complains more about my snoring when I have put on a couple of extra pounds. When I take that weight off…the snoring decreases!!! Allergy problems may also affect the way that you sleep. Congested sinuses make breathing difficult. This will greatly affect the soundness of your sleep.

WHAT SHOULD I BE TAKING?

❑ Calcium—You need about 1200 mg a day, spread throughout the day. For FMS patients, I also recommend taking an extra 500 mg at bedtime. Now there has been a lot of hoopla about getting calcium from taking an antacid tablet. That is just stupid. Sorry. The fact is, when you study calcium absorption, you find that in order for calcium to be absorbed, it must be absorbed in an acidic environment. According their own ads, the tablets "neutralize" stomach acids!! See why eating a handful of antacid tablets to get your calcium just doesn't make sense!! You don't have to be a rocket scientist to figure this out! My brother, Dr. J. Michael Weir, once wrote in his newspaper column that "Taking an antacid for the calcium is like drinking a martini to get the vitamin C in the olive!" in other words, just take your calcium supplement and be done with it!

❑ Magnesium. I believe a greater problem than a calcium deficiency is the magnesium deficiency. If you don't have calcium, then magnesium cannot be absorbed by the body. So, if you have a magnesium deficiency, you will automatically have a magnesium deficiency. I have searched the world over, and finally came up with my own formula. It is called "RELAX" It is powdered magnesium that turns into a liquid when you add hot water. This product is almost miraculous! I added vitamin C, Potassium, Zinc and MSM to the magnesium. I recommend drinking it right before going to bed. People will usually tell me that they had their best night of sleep ever after drinking this. Why liquid? Anytime that you can take a mineral in liquid form, it is utilized by the body almost immediately. There is no pill breakdown in order for it to be absorbed…it is already ready to be absorbed.

Try the Relax FIRST!   If you notice that you need some further help, then add ONE of the following!
❑   Valerian Root. This is a great root, with a beautiful gentle sleep as the side effect. Does it work for everyone? No!   But I recommend trying it. Start with one capsule about one hour before going to bed. It is worth the try.
❑   Melatonin. This naturally occurring hormone helps the body regulate its normal sleep cycles. These can get off kilter after long trips, working a weird schedule, or being unable to sleep for other reasons. By the time we reach forty, the body has significantly slowed its production of melatonin and so by the time we're sixty-five, production is down by more than half. If you lay there for hours, staring at the ceiling before sleep comes, try melatonin.   But how much?   That's the million dollar question. I recommend no more than 6 mg. Start out with 1 mg for a few nights, and if that's not enough to improve your sleep, keep increasing by 1 mg until you reach 6 mg.   If 6 mg doesn't help, then perhaps you are one of the few who will not respond to melatonin.   Now here is an interesting side effect in a certain percentage of the population…NIGHTMARES! Yes, some patients who take this product get terrible nightmares! Listen, you already have enough problems sleeping without dreaming about your husband gouging your eyes out with a garden hoe! Worth the try? You bet!
❑   L-Tryptophan. This is a great product. Does it work great? Yes, in some people. Take it with the

same instructions that are given for melatonin, but only go up to 4 mg. Be careful with this product, because you cannot take it if you are on an SSRI!!!

RELAX FORMULA
One of the greatest things I have done in my career is to come up with this formula. It is a combination of Magesium, Vitamin D and MSM. If you read above, you will see the incredible need for Magnesium. But not just magnesium. As with most pills, when you take them....they break down so slowly that the body has a hard time using them. That's why I have made this formula to be taken as a drink. It comes in a powder and when added to hot water, turns to a drink. The key to this is...it begins absorbing IN YOUR MOUTH!!! There is an almost immediate reaction by your body. Then I added Vitamin D. As you know, you just don't get enough! I wish that everyone would get out in the sun at least 20 minutes every day without sunscreen, but it doesn't happen. Again, you are going to have to take some form of supplement. This form is in the powder that turns to liquid. Finally, we add in MSM. This is a short, quick name for methyl-sufonyl-methane. If you have heard of DMSO, this is what is known as a metabolite of DMSO. It is an organic form of sulfur again that naturally is in the body, but deficient in quantity.
We have used just enough to help the body over some of these rough spots.

Don't try to reinvent the wheel. It took us a long time to get the right balance between all of these, and then in a form that the body can use. Stop reading this right now....yes you heard me. Go to

your computer and go to my website at
www.TheFirstChoiceLife.com or
www.RelaxFormula.com and order some. You will
be amazed at the immediate difference you feel.
You cannot get this at health food stores or online
any place else.   This is a Dr. Weir original. Believe
me, you will be kissing my feet in days!!

IRRITABLE BOWEL SYNDROME

"Doc, I'm so tired of having the runs, I don't know what to do!" I hear that statement all the time from my patients. If this happens frequently to you, more than likely you are dealing with IBS. This gastrointestinal problem hits the large intestine like the Marines hit Normandy and because it is inflammatory in nature, it will leave you wrung out.

Irritable bowel syndrome may take the form of either diarrhea or constipation, and accompanying it will be abdominal pain, gas, bloating, and mucous in the stool. It's caused by the same muscular tension that creates all those pain flare-ups elsewhere. The intestines, after all, are simply bands of muscles through which digested good is moved, then eliminated as waste.

A practical word of warning; while you are in a healing phase, give your body a break! Switch to a more bland diet and skip the tacos and enchiladas, salsa and Texas Pete! Bland foods will help your intestinal tract heal much faster. Because there is such a large allergic reaction to wheat with FMS patients, eliminating this from your diet will help this condition greatly. If you have suffered with this, then I highly recommend having a full workup done, including cancer screening. Better safe, than sorry.

You Want Me To Stick That WHERE?

I am also a big proponent of retention enemas for this condition. There is often a loss of the good bacteria in the intestinal tract. This is especially true if you have taken a lot of antibiotics over the years. An easy way to replace these, is to take an enema with acidophilus in the water. L. Bifidus is what you are looking for. Go to a health food store and buy a good acidophilus product. The best are in the refrigerated section. There are several forms, Eugalen Topfer Forte is considered one of the best for this procedure. You are going to take about 2-8 ounces of the acidophilus, and put it into one quart of warm (NOT HOT!) distilled water. Mix this very well, until it is dissolved in the water. You are going to put that in the enema bag, and implant this into the colon. You certainly don't want me to draw another one of my pictures like the tender point picture for this section….so go online for instructions on how to do an enema. You want to retain this in the colon for up to one hour. Sometimes people will have to take an enema with just plain distilled water first (not retention)…to get some of the fecal material out first. Believe me, the first couple times you will not be able to hold it for an hour…but practice makes perfect. This is great if you are suffering from a lot of gas and mucus. I recommend that you only do these once every 2 months. (6 times per year)

I recommend the following herbs and vitamins to help relieve this painful condition:
❑ ALOE VERA JUICE. Drink from one-half to cone cup of this healthful concoction three times a day on an empty stomach. It has great healing powers for the mucous membranes, and it is also

good for ulcers. You will find this at a health food store. Now days, they even have flavored juices.

❑ ALFALFA TABLETS. Take one capsule three times a day, with meals. This helps to replenish vitamin K in the body. This will also help digestion, and keep intestinal flora healthy and happy!

❑ ACIDOPHILUS. You will usually find these capsules on the refrigerated shelves of your health food stores. Take these as directed, and make sure that you store these in your refrigerator. I also recommend eating a good wholesome cultured yogurt with your breakfast. Please understand me…this is not the flavored yogurt that you get at the local grocery store. This is a good yogurt that is purchased at a health food store. This is one time that you can sweeten it with some honey. This is also great mixed with a natural granola. This is immensely important for building up the intestinal flora!

❑ FIBER. A particularly good source of fiber may be either oat or rice bran. It helps regulate bowel movements and will not leave you dragged out as some laxatives do. Have this at breakfast with some yogurt, maybe some "fresh" berries on top.

❑ CHARCOAL TABLETS. These can be found at a health food store and they will help to absorb excess gas. If you experience a "Rumbly in your Tumbly," then these may be your life-savers! Take five to six of these little puppies whenever you feel gas symptoms. Please don't use these everyday, because they also absorb some vital nutrients. As with all of these products…don't overdo them!

❑ PEPPERMINT OIL TEA. This wonderful, soothing drink helps calm down the intestinal tract.

If you eat and feel bloated and full fast, try some of this tea—with a little honey, if you must. It will give almost instant results.

MUSCLE CRAMPS AND ACHES! It's when the leg muscles cramp up or you get that jittery feeling in your legs. Sometimes it may last all night, greatly contributing to your sleep disorder. Therefore, it's important that you get this situation under control ASAP.

It's important that you again make sure this condition of muscle cramps and aches is properly distinguished from other problems, such as "intermittent claudication"—a disorder that affects blood flow to the legs. Check that out with your physician. If you tend to cramp after you walk, but get relief when you stop, then you may be suffering from intermittent claudication. If your physician, after examining you, finds that you don't have it, what you are probably dealing with is the kind of cramping associated with FMS.

Another common condition that is gaining more notice day by day is a condition known as RLS-Restless Leg Syndrome. This is where the legs just don't want to be held still. You lay there at night, and it either feels like grasshoppers are crawling all over your legs, or you have jittery spasms in them so they will not lay still. Regardless, I am recommending the following things for you to consider:

❑ CALCIUM—Again, you want at least 1200 mg per day. Take this at night before you go to bed. Don't forget though, it is usually a magnesium deficiency that is more the problem than calcium...so..

❑ MAGNESIUM. I cannot impress upon you enough the importance of getting this mineral in your body. I have had several people who have literally come back from the brink of death with just this! I'm going to tell you again that the RELAX FORMULA I have put together is your key. This will make the world of difference in how you feel.

❑ VITAMIN E. This great antioxidant helps increase circulation in the extremities. If you aren't taking it now, start immediately. If you aren't taking it now, start immediately—but start out slow. Start with 400 IU per day, for two weeks, increasing another 400 IU daily for two weeks, and then add another 400 IU daily until you reach 1200 IU per day. This is your maximum dose. It is important for you to be taking this vitamin if you are taking fish oils!

❑ POTASSIUM. Vital for leg cramping and achy muscles. I recommend about 100 mg per day. Potassium is important, especially in relation to calcium and magnesium. Now you have heard the old adage, "An apple a day, keeps the doctor away"…switch fruits! "A banana a day…"

❑ Coenzyme Q10. Heart function improves, as does circulation with the addition of this supplement. Take 100-120 mg per day. I have heard many patients comment that their blood pressure also decreased when they began to take Q10. Some renowned cardiologists have stated the importance of Q10 with magnesium in the prevention of heart problems. If you have a family history of heart disease, then this is one thing you don't want to be without!

❑ FOLIC ACID. I am recommending this for you if you have RLS. This is an incredible vitamin for a properly functioning nervous system. You will find that this also will help with depression. I recommend that you take this together with Vitamin B12.

LOW ENERGY

If you feel like a washed out old rage by the end of the day, regardless of how much sleep you seem to get, perhaps it's not just sleep that you need, but a change in diet and dietary supplements. If you feel like you've been run over by an entire fleet of Mack trucks on a cross-country marathon, maybe it's your body telling you that it's time to make some changes.

The greatest help in your quest to reduce fatigue will be the introduction of a low-carbohydrate diet. High-carbohydrate foods will keep that rollercoaster effect going indefinitely, since all that sugar gives you a sudden burst of energy, followed by a crash. Don't let that sudden burst of energy fool you. It is a pseudo energy. Imagine taking your blood sugar up to a high, getting a rush, then all of a sudden for no reason the "feel-good" rush is gone, sending your blood sugar level crashing to the floor. If you do that everyday, no wonder you feel washed out. Get on some good protein and stay away from those refined carbs. You'll be glad you did. You know I'm talking to you if your desk drawer has 32 varieties of candy bars stuffed in it. How about some peanut butter or cheese as an afternoon snack instead?

Then add these things to your diet:

❑   IRON. Because the blood carries the iron so needed by your body, it's important to make sure that you're getting enough. The problem with getting iron into the system, is that iron pills just don't work. I can't tell you how many times over the years we have x-rayed patients, and seen the iron pills following the intestines out the back door! Another problem is that they can cause constipation.

Now, this may sound crazy, but a great source of iron is gained by using a cast iron skillet when you cook. The heat releases small amount of iron from the skillet, and it is mixed with your food. Just the residual iron from that skillet is enough for you on a daily basis. Another great source of iron is molasses. Now I'm not talking about the sugar sweet, refined molasses that you get at your local grocery store. I'm talking about some good old-fashioned blackstrap molasses. This can still be purchased at a good whole-foods market or health food store. Take a couple of teaspoons of this a couple of times per week. Finally, if you have a good health food store, many of them will sell a Dessicated Liver tablet. These tablets will help to boost your energy. This is much easier than frying up liver in the skillet. The thing about the dessicated liver tablets, is that they have been "cleaned up" so that none of the toxins found in regular liver are not present. Remember, that the liver is the detoxifier of the blood. It cleans out all the toxins in the blood, and when you fry it up and eat it…you're getting everything! I mean everything!

❑ Bee Pollen. Don't go overboard! Just a tiny amount on the end of a spoon is enough to start with, building up to two teaspoons per day. This is a great energy booster that won't crash you later. Royal Bee Jelly is also very good.

❑ SIBERIAN GINSING. This is a great natural energy booster. Try it around noontime to help you through that afternoon "drop." It comes in liquid or capsule form, but the liquid form absorbs quicker.

❑ SPIRULINA. A good source of protein, spirulina also increases energy and can be taken in capsule or powder form. I like to mix a scoop of spirulina with a couple cups of rice dream, ½ of a banana, strawberries and ice in a blender. WOW! This is a great "pick me up" snack. This makes a great breakfast shake for people who are on the run!

DEPLETED ADRENALS

This really goes under the energy portion, but I feel that it deserves some extra attention. These tiny glands located just on top of the kidneys are not to be underestimated. Also called our "fight or flight" glands, the adrenals produce the hormone epinephrine, which is also called adrenalin. That's the hormone released when we're in stress...and FMS patients certainly qualify for that category.

Adrenalin is what gives us the power to stay and fight or turn in fright. Problem is…our stress-filled society constantly causes the adrenal glands to pump so hard, they can become depleted. When that happens, it is common to feel fatigue and adrenal deficiency. Another common symptom of this condition is a dull headache.

There is an easy test to check for depleted adrenal glands. Get a blood pressure cuff (one of the new digital ones works best) and lay down on your bed, taking your blood pressure while laying down. Then stand up, and immediately retake your blood pressure. It should be ten points higher than laying down. If it does not go up, or if it decreases, you may suspect the adrenals are depleted.

There are a couple of things that you need to try if the above test is positive:

❑ ADRENERGY. This is a product from Morter Health Products. This booster will do a lot to increase energy and stamina. It's a combination of raw adrenal gland and specialized herbs that actually helps to health and refurbish the adrenal glands. The key to this product is that it helps take some of the stress off the adrenal glands until they can recoup! If you can't find Adrenergy, ask your health food store for an adrenal support product.

Editors Note; do not take Adrenergy while pregnant. It is vital for expectant mothers to stay at an even keel without any major fluctuations in the hormones, especially adrenalin.

❑ DESSICATED LIVER. This is important to help support the liver, another adrenal function. Made from liver that has been purified, it comes in capsule form. Take as directed and you will notice an increase in energy level.

❑ MILK THISTLE/SILYMARIN. This is also good for the liver and adrenal glands, and helpful in the treatment of liver dysfunction and cirrhosis. It is also helpful to bring healing to liver damage due to drug usage. Taking this product may cause loose stools, since it wakes up the liver and increases bile flow. I recently had a nurse who was having problems after being diagnosed with hepatitis. Her complexion was constantly filled with blemishes because of the toxins built up from a faulty liver. She was amazed after we put her on milk thistle. It really makes a difference.

❑ ASTRAGALUS. This herb helps improve adrenal gland function and helps you deal with stress. You can purchase it at your local health food store. Take as directed on the label. This is a great friend to help you defeat fatigue.

HEADACHES/MIGRAINES

If all the other bothersome symptoms of FMS were not enough, you get headaches. Because you have FMS, you already feel bad all over. The migraine is the icing on the cake. Whether frontal, temporal, or sub-occipital (back of the head), these severe, banging headaches can bring much pain and discomfort. The typical migraine often begins with a full, throbbing pain behind one or both of the eyes. One of the text book signs of migraines, is the presence of an "aura"—that feeling of being in the twilight zone…flashing lights…sparklers going off…out of touch with reality. Some even experience a type of tunnel vision where peripheral vision is lost.

Headaches like these can be quite scary. I remember having migraines as a child and holding my hand six inches in front of my face and not being able to see it. The visual problems were so severe that I could not see my hand, let alone 6 feet in front of me! These visual side-effects are very commonly associated with migraine headaches.

I hate to be the bearer of more bad news, but caffeine, including chocolate, is a precipitator of headaches. It's what's known as a "trigger" and can set off a migraine in a heartbeat. With the presence of FMS, it doesn't take much to trigger a migraine, so keep caffeine intake to a minimum and avoid it altogether if you can.

It is interesting to note that many patients experience some relief from migraines after vomiting. Afterwards, the headache seems to subside. Apparently vomiting helps to release some of the pressure and assists the body in dealing with the migraine.

Here's a trick I recommend: Try what I call the "Switch-a-roo technique." Start with two towels, one doused in hot water, the other doused in ice water. Place the hot towel on the forehead and the cold towel on the back of the neck. Keep these in place for about 10 minutes. Then switch. Drench the towels again, one in hot water and the other in cold water, and switch their locations. Place the hot towel on the neck, and the iced towel on the forehead. Continue switching for about an hour, alternating towels from hot to cold and cold to hot. You will notice that the headache will begin to subside. But make sure the hot towels are not steaming…you don't want blisters.

Also, try one or more of these excellent sources of relief:

❑   FEVERFEW

This is not an instant cure, but over time it helps. This herb not only helps to relieve headaches, but its long-range benefits are tremendous. It contains the same qualities as aspirin in helping to reduce secretion of inflammatory particles from platelets and white blood cells. It helps migraines because of the serotonin released by the platelets, which cause blood vessels to spasm. Many people notice a decrease in the intensity and frequency of migraines, once they start on this product. But don't try it for two weeks and then give up!! Stay with it and you will notice eventual results, even if they are not measurable until five or six months of steady use! I recommend 25 mg, twice a day.

CHIROPRACTIC

There are two things that chiropractors have become famous for treating over the years. Number one is lower back pain, number two is headaches. I cannot tell you how many times a patient walks in with a migraine and walks out without one!! The problem is, a lot of chiropractors get too heavy handed. They are Sumu Wrestlers on the weekends. I love using the Pro-Adjuster on patients because the results can be almost immediate. It is a completely safe form of therapy. Go to www.Pro-Adjuster.us and find a chiropractor near you that uses this technique! Another great low force technique is the Activator. This is the granddaddy of them all. I used it for a number of years, and the results are great. You can check them out at www.Activator.com.

THYROID

Something that I did not address much in the first edition of this book was the thyroid gland. This little gland, located at the front of the neck, can cause a multitude of problems if it is out of balance or not working. It is so important for you to have blood tests to check for hypothyroidism. Find a doctor that is willing to check this out for you.

Oh my darlin, Oh my darlin, Oh my darlin Iodine…..

I was totally amazed when I first began to test patients for Iodine deficiencies. It blew me out of the water. I began to look at patients with pain in the trapezius muscles along the base of the neck, patients with headaches, and people with brain fatigue. Of course, we knew that this was present in the patients with hypothyroidism, but when we began to broaden that search out, the changes were phenomenal. I remember having a nurse that worked in our clinic that woke up every morning with headaches. It was like clockwork. I cannot imagine starting every day like that, but she did. So, we did our 24 hour iodine test on her. Guess what? She was deficient in iodine, and within 3 days of starting taking the supplements, she was headache free!

Let's start with this indepth, difficult 24 hour iodine test. Are you ready? Go to Walgreens, and get a small bottle of iodine. Yes, the orange liquid in the small bottle that your mother used to dab on sores.

You know, the one you spilled on the bathroom sink, and it stained it. Now, you want to paint a patch of this on your forearm, about the size of a silver dollar. You have to understand this fact; this patch should remain on the arm for about 48 hours. So, start this in the morning after your shower. Paint it on your arm, and then every ½ hour, check to see if it is still there. If it is gone before 12 hours, then you have a severe deficiency. If it is 24 hours, a moderate deficiency, and anything less than 48 hours is mild. How do you correct this? Take iodine. If you have a severe deficiency, you are going to have to take about 50mg per day. That is a lot. You cannot get this much from eating salt either…you would have to eat 10 pounds of it per day. You must be faithful with this. It will take about 8-12 months to rebuild that iodine storehouse. Then, once a month, do another iodine test. Once it stays there for 48 hours, then you are ok.

As a matter of aesthetics, you may want to paint this on your belly, so it doesn't show on your arm. Please wait until it dries fully, before you get dressed or you may have an orange circle painted on all your blouses or shirts.

What in the world is Selenium?

Selenium is a mineral. It is an incredible part of
your health and well-being. It was discovered that
sheep and cattle in New Zealand were suffering
from muscular breakdown because of the low levels
of selenium in the soils there. As the diet was
changed, the muscular breakdown was halted. Not
only does this affect skeletal muscle, but it also
affects cardiac muscles. This is a powerful
antioxidant.

I recommend taking this mineral with your vitamin
D and E. This is a mineral that is found in
broccoli, chicken, diary, liver, onions, seafood and
certain vegetables. Again, the easiest way is to find
it in capsular form. Simply take the label
directions.

VITAMIN D

I'm always looking for something that will help the Fibromyalgia patient, and the hottest thing off of the press is this....Vitamin D. As you know, Vitamin D is a fat-soluble vitamin. It is extremely important in the absorption of calcium into the system. Without it...you will have a calcium deficiency and all of the ramifications that accompany that! What we are also finding, is that it is the most deficient vitamin in the body of people with Fibromyalgia.

We have come through a phase, especially in America, where if you went outside without any type of sunscreen, you felt like you were naked. The problem with this is, without the sun rays, there chemical reaction to produce Vitamin D is greatly hindered. Am I saying go without sunscreen? Not necessarily. But I also believe that it is good just to get out in the warm sun for a couple of minutes everyday without slathering on buckets of the latest SFP lotion. Don't overdo it! As with everything...use wisdom. But feeling the warmth of the sun rays can be quite calming.

Now, how much Vitamin D should you take? If you have Fibromyalgia, then I would recommend 5,000 to 10,000 IU per day. I highly recommend that you take this with your calcium and magnesium. I also recommend that you take some vitamin E with this also...400-1200 IU per day. Here's my prescription...get some sun and take your Vitamin D.

"But the cats are following me home...."
You have already heard me talk about fish oils...but
it bears repeating...you weren't listening before!!!
I will never forget when someone told me to take
Fish Oil capsules...I tasted them....and I just knew
that cats would start following me home.   When I
first started to take them years ago, they were not as
"savvy" as they are now.   Now they come "Enteric
Coated," so that they don't start to dissolve until
after they hit the intestinal area.   Regardless, these
are an incredible part of the FMS patients' regimen.

If you do a full study of how the body reacts to what
we eat, you will find that the Essential Fatty Acids
play a huge role in decreasing inflammation in the
body. These little buggers are tremendous aids in
brain function.   Remember the short-term memory
loss?   Oh yeah! It is my opinion that these EFA's
are right on the front lines of your defense against
arthritis, skin conditions, breast cancer and nerve
integrity.   All of these are important in the battle
against Fibromyalgia.   There is much discussion
over how to get these into your system...Primrose
oil, black currant seed oil or Fish Oil.   My opinion
is that Fish Oil is the best.   The deep, cold-water
fish provide the best sources of EPA oils.   Where
there is concern about toxicity found in the fish oils,
just make sure that you buy a product that has been
screened for these. There has been a lot of hoopla
over the mercury in fish oil...and it is just
that...hoopla.   The only people that should not take
Fish oils are diabetic patients.   Otherwise...Fish on.
How much?   I take 8-10 capsules per day.

As a side note, the fish oils are absolutely incredible
for children. If you have a child that suffers from

learning problems, then there is no doubt…they need to be taking the fish oils. I recommend 1-3 per day for them. There are unbelievable changes in behavior with these. I also use these for patients with mood disorders. I recommend 10-20 per day for these folks. You will see immediate changes in behavior. You know me…any time that you can stay away from psych meds….the better off you are.

I am also recommending that you take vitamin E with these pills. 400-1200 IU per day when you take these.

Finally, when you first start to take these, you may burp up a fishy "aftertaste." Sometimes what some patients do is to freeze their capsules before they take them, and this often eliminates that aftertaste. Kinda like a frozen fish stick!!
Actually, take these, and then a little mayonnaise and some pickle relish and you have yourself a little snack! Only kidding!

Go to our website and you will find the Fish Oils that I take. I am rather particular on these. I want the cleanest and best for myself and my family and now for you.

THIRTEEN

Just take a bath…and other fabulous advice!

Now hold on! What can taking a bath have to do to help all those finicky FMS symptoms? More than you realize!   Why not use my recipe for a relaxing warm bath and get therapeutic results too?

First realize that your achy muscles are craving attention.   They are literally gasping for oxygen, so we need to look for ways to increase oxygen both internally and externally. An easy way to do that is to soak in a nice tube of hot water containing things that heal.   First, take two cups of apple cider vinegar and two cups of Epsom salts, and let them dissolve together in a tub of hot water.   Put the kids to bed, put on some relaxing music, light a couple of scented candles climb into the tub, and soak. Don't answer the phone. Don't read. Don't do anything but relax.   This is your time, and your muscles will thank you for it all night long.   As soon as you are fully relaxed and your bath is finished…go to bed.   This combination of apple cider vinegar and Epsom salts creates Malic acid, which is miraculous with FMS.

If you are one of those people that love electric blankets…sell them!!   If you want to warm up the bed…turn them on, and then take them off right before you lay down.   The electric blanket wires creates an electrical field that interferes with your bodies own electrical field. It can confuse your body and interfere with sleep.   In winter, use the good old-fashioned flannel sheets.   These can be purchased at most department stores and will keep warmth in!! Plus, they just feel great next to the skin, which is always therapeutic.

Let me offer some advice on a few other topics before we part company, knowing that FMS patients may also have trouble with hormonal imbalance, weight and sinuses. Let's not leave anything out.

HORMONE IMBALANCE

I have seen a number of causes for hormone imbalance. In the case of one of my patients, a breast biopsy was performed with complications, and started many of her problems. Whatever the cause, we must work at getting those hormone levels restored as quickly as possible. These chemicals are simply encoded message carriers that turn certain systems on and off. They tell the body's systems what to do and when to do it. Throw this off, and you'll wind up with major problems as these messages start getting messed up.

Do you have hormonal issues?

A friend sent this to me….do these fit you?

ESTROGEN ISSUES:

10 ways to know if you have Estrogen issues:

1. Everyone around you has an attitude problem.
2. You're adding chocolate chips to your cheese omelet.
3. The dryer has shrunk every last pair of your jeans.
4. Your husband is suddenly agreeing to everything that you say.
5. You're using your cellular phone to dial up every bumper sticker that says: "How's my driving? Call 1-800….
6. Everyone's head looks like an invitation to batting practice
7. Everyone seems to have just landed here from "Outer Space"
8. The cat makes more sense than your husband.
9. You're sure that everyone is scheming to drive you crazy.
10. The Ibuprofen bottle is empty and you just bought it yesterday!

Is this you? We need to talk. A friend of mine told me he was worried about suicide with his wife who suffered from menopause…he was more worried about HOMICIDE!

First of all, clean up your diet. Stop eating garbage. Your body is already in a state of shock due to FMS and imbalanced hormones. It needs all the help it can get, so don't keep on dumping in sugar and carbs. Your body needs to be reeled back in from Mars.

Second, women should begin the use of progesterone cream. This cream brings many benefits including improved brain function, diminished muscular aches, improved skin problems, and improved sleep patterns. Certain women who complained of loss of libido also noted improvement with the use of this cream.

Progesterone cream is simply rubbed on the body and is an effective way to restore progesterone levels naturally.   It is derived from the Mexican Wild yam root.

Women will notice incredible changes after using this cream. I have heard the husbands of some of my patients refer to it as "that magic cream". Many men would sell their boats to buy this for their wives.

WEIGHT LOSS

Many of us need to lose some weight. But FMS patients should pay special attention to losing the weight they need to lose, since excess weight only compounds the pain and discomfort of this disease. How do you lose weight when you already feel so rotten?

I've heard comments like these a million times: "Doc, I just can't lose weight. I seem to walk by food and put on ten pounds. Help!" Excess weight is a very difficult issue for people because it can damage their self-esteem. The problem with FMS patients is that it is really harder for them to lose, since it's difficult for them to exercise and that adds more weight...and when you add more weight, it makes it more difficult to exercise...you get the picture?

I have tried it all! I have eaten that prepackaged food that tasted like cardboard. I have tried the ground up chalk milkshakes, been on the fad starvation diets, and taken enough prescription weight loss medications to be as skinny as a rail. I've counted calories, fat grams, carbs, the number of bites you chew...you name it...I've tried it.

Let me give you a little secret I discovered. Somewhere in my history, I made a decision to gain weight. There was someone or something that I discovered that I wanted to be like, and I made that decision. Do some meditation, and discover where in your history you made that decision.

Secondly, find a program that fits your lifestyle, and get some help. South Beach diet, Atkins, Sugar Busters, Weight Watchers are a couple. It is amazing how much we eat and justify eating!! To be honest, we really are never hungry!! The fact is, if you eat the right things, you body will not crave them as much. Because when you crave them, you have to eat and eat and eat trying to help satisfy those deficiencies. If the truth be told, if you would cut out all wheat from your diet, and SUGAR…you would automatically lose weight without paying someone to tell you some stupid stuff to keep you coming!

There is no one thing that can cause a gain in weight. Most people look at someone overweight and they are thinking…"If they would get off their fat behinds and quit eating so much, they wouldn't be so fat". Folks, if it were that easy, nobody would be overweight! 99% of these people are dealing with something in their body that is causing this problem. Do you know how frustrating it is to be on a diet, and yet not lose anything? Believe me, it is frustration to the nth degree!! Let me give you a Readers Digest version of what I believe are the main villains:

FOOD ALLERGY. If there is something that you are allergic to, and don't know it, it can throw your entire system off so that you put weight on. Find someone who can test you for food allergies. (check with a chiropractor who does muscle testing)
THYROID. If you have a problem with the thyroid gland, you will not be able to lose weight. The body is out of balance, and it is trying to survive.
SLEEP APNEA. In the bodies fight to stay alive at night, there is extra pressure put on certain organs and glands. When these are stimulated, the body is not able to lose weight.
CANDITA OVERGROWTH. Put in simple terms, this is an overgrowth of yeast in the body. We see this a lot with people who have taken a lot of

antibiotics over the years. This will show up as fatigue, memory loss and an inability to lose weight.

First thing to do is to make sure that your doctor has checked you for all of these things. Take the appropriate steps to combat each issue, an then move on with life. Does this mean that you can eat anything that you want to? No. But it does mean that when you put out the effort to lose the weight, your body will respond correctly, and you will lose weight. Imagine for a minute if you had all four of those things above. Wow, what a battle! Can you also see that you can have more than one thing causing your weight gain, and just cutting calories is not going to help! You MUST find the causes of your problem and correct them.

SINUS PROBLEMS

Believe it or not, many times sinus problems are actually triggered by the use of dairy products. Cut them out, and you will notice immediate results. You may even notice a reduction in body pain. Several of my patients get severe neck pain when the sinuses are involved. Sinus congestion can also cause severe headaches, post-nasal drip and sore throats.

First, we remove the triggers. The number one biggest producer of mucus?????? SOY! Yes you heard that right. Not only does this product mess up your hormonal system, it will produce more mucus than you ever wanted. That will start to build up in the sinus cavities and you end up with all kinds of trouble. Aren't you glad you bought this book....just for that one fact. That also means getting off all dairy products, which are merely composed of mucous from cows. Yet we drink milk as if it were the staff of life. Humans are the only living creatures who continue to drink milk once they are weaned from it...and then it is not even the milk from our own species. That is sick. Can you imagine an adult cow doing the same? But we drink gallons of the stuff because the ads on TV tell us that it's good for us, and we believe them. We are already dealing with a physical problem that stems from the accumulation of mucous, so we add more fuel to the fire. We add more mucous to a body that has already demonstrated that it cannot deal with the mucous that it has. That doesn't make sense...does it?

I recommend staying away from dairy products like milk, cheese and ice cream. These are the main offenders. Cottage cheese and yogurt seem to be fine because they are cultured.

"But how am I going to get my calcium?" you ask. My answer is simple…Not from dairy products. These products are no longer rich in calcium as in our grandparents' day. Today, milk producers pasteurize, homogenize, and agonize the milk until there is no longer any redeeming value in terms of calcium content. We haven't even touched on the hormones given to the cows that cause the milk production to increase. Ever wonder why little Jenny down the street has breasts at the age of 12 that you didn't get until you were 22? Instead, eat green leafy vegetables. They're loaded with calcium.

I would be remiss if I didn't walk about something that has come up with my patients over and over. Is there really a difference between magnesium in a pill and liquid magnesium, and the answer is YES! I have had so many patients over the years who have been taking magnesium in a pill, and when I talk to them about magnesium deficiency, they tell me that they are already taking it…in a pill. But the fact is, they still show all of the symptoms of a magnesium deficiency. The fact is, if your body is not absorbing whatever you take…it doesn't do you any good to take it! I hate to beat a dead horse…but why spend money on something that isn't going to do you any good. It's like having a hole in the ground, and thinking that you have it covered, when you really don't! You walk out in the yard and fall into the hole…"Well, that hole is covered!" No, you just think it is. This goes along with people who buy their vitamins from those cheap discount mail order catalogs…you know…3 bottles of vitamins for .99 cents, plus you get a FREE oxygenated hair brush with your order. I don't know about you, but I think that I'm worth the extra cost to get something that my body is really going to use. I recently had one of our employees have a test for the blood levels of her magnesium, and to her amazement, her blood levels were showing as low. The fact is, she had been taking the pill form of magnesium for years! Did she switch to liquid right away? Yes she did. The fact is, the liquid form of magnesium is assimilated into the body almost immediately, starting in the mucous membranes of the mouth. Within minutes, you will feel the calming effects in your body.

What are some of the symptoms of a magnesium deficiency? Let me give them to you:
FATIGUE
DEPRESSION
MUSCLE PAIN
CARDIAC PROBLEMS
INSOMNIA
PMS
HORMONE INBALANCE
HEADACHES
MUSCLE SPASMS AND CRAMPS
ABNORMAL HEART RHYTHMS
IRRITABILITY
NERVOUSNESS
ANXIOUSNESS

Any of these sound familiar? Take my word for it…if you are reading this book, you need to get some as soon as possible. Go to my website and

check it out right now.   Your body is screaming for
you to get started.

"I keeping walking into the door frame!"
I just heard it again this week.   "Dr. Weir, I don't
know what is wrong with me…I keep walking into
the door frame! I feel like I can't walk a straight
line."   It is amazing with this disease, comes a host
of other irritating little gnomes.   One of these is a
loss of balance and the desire to "list" to one side or
another. The problem with this is, you tend to "list"
to the side when you are going in a certain
direction.   "I feel like a klutz!"   Well, you are!
Just kidding. The fact is, you cannot control that.
You have built into you a mechanism for keeping
you upright and steering in the right direction.
When that mechanism gets off, your body loses that
control. A wrench gets thrown into your system,
and you have problems in your "Cross-Crawl
Pattern".   WHAT IS THAT?   That is the system in
your brain that sends impulses from one side to the
other.   When that gets out of whack…you lean to
one side or the other. This pattern starts when you
are a baby. As you begin to crawl, it sets that
system into place. Then when you stand and walk,
it is a normal thing for you to do.
    PROBLEM NUMBER ONE: We don't always
allow kids to crawl. We are worried if they aren't
walking by a certain age, so we are so quick to grab

them by the hands and make them walk. QUIT IT!
Let your baby crawl around the house. Don't be in
such a rush. When they do, they are establishing
their "Cross-Crawl Pattern." That is so incredibly
important. We often get into a contest with the
neighbors over how fast our kids do certain things.
My God...let them grow at their own rates.

What does that have to do with you? If you find
yourself running into door frames, then you need to
Re-establish your Cross Crawl Pattern. How do
you do that? CRAWLING! You better believe it.
I recommend the first thing in the morning, before
you stand on your feet, get on your hands and
knees. Simply crawl around your bedroom. Do it
for 4-5 minutes. I recommend getting up before
anyone else in the house, so that they don't see you
and have ammunition for a later "ribbing". You
will be amazed at the difference this simple thing
makes.

T.M.J.

This is not a new James Bond Movie! These three little letters can cause more problems than you could imagine. They stand for Temporal Mandibular Joint. Put it simply…your jaw joint. This puppy can throw you into more pain than you ever thought possible. WOW. I'm serious. When this little joint gets roused, it makes life a living hell. If you find that you are having serious problems with this, then you need to find a chiropractor that uses either the Activator Methods technique or the Pro-Adjuster Technique and have them check you out. You may have to try mouth pieces and some other things too. You want to stay away from any type of surgical intervention as much as possible. It can start as a clicking in the jaw joint, to severe pain when chewing. A common problem with FMS patients. Take my advice, have a chiropractic exam to start with!

FOURTEEN

You Better Learn to Laugh!

If you are around me very long, you are going to find that I don't take anything too seriously. I have discovered that life is way to short, and if you spend the entire time seriously trying to discover the meaning of life, you missed it. I have come to the conclusion that from the moment you slide out the mommy shoot, to the moment they lay your head on the satin pillow, you simply have millions of moments to create the life that you want. I am amazed by the people who are so concerned that every move they make be in the "perfect will of God" and He is looking at them waiting for them to make a move. The fact of the matter is, you have been created in the image of God, and He is a creator. Your greatest gift is the ability to create. You have been placed where you are with tremendous talents and abilities. You have gifts inside of you yet untapped. Use them to create. Quit saying how it could have been, or should have been and make it be what you want it to be. But quit being so serious about it.

When is the last time that you went to a comedy movie and just laughed? When is the last time that you laughed so hard at a joke that milk came out your nose? Are you more concerned about what other people think about what you may do…or are you doing it because you love to do it? My prescription to you is to go out and rent a funny movie and just sit and laugh. You will quickly realize that all of the important things to you soon become less important. Take time to stop and enjoy the ride. I remember as a kid going on a long road trip. Whenever we would see something fun along the way, my dad would pull over. It took us longer to get to where we were going, but guess what? It made the entire trip more enjoyable and memorable. I look at the way some people live their lives and realize that they think the end is their destination. They don't realize that the entire journey is what is to be enjoyed. Some people are so careful….afraid to do anything in life. They want to make sure that they make it safely to death!!! Guess what? It is time to break out of the mold. Get wild. Do things that you have wanted to but were afraid that people would judge you for. Jesh! Put on your dancing shoes, buy a microphone, sing in the rain, buy some Play dough, ask for a kids menu while you are waiting for your food and color it…play the games on it, wear clothes that you like to wear, turn up the stereo and listen to Bon Jovi, or just sit in front of a fireplace with the love of your life and drink a glass of wine and kiss the night away. It's time to live!

Norm Cousins
Read his story. He survived a serious illness by watching comedies. Get some of those old movies and t.v. shows. Carol Burnette shows are a great example. She is funny. I love Chevy Chase. Just

get about 10 of them and have someone keep the kids, get some great snacks and lock yourself in the bedroom to laugh. The great thing about those old shows is that they are good clean fun.

EPILOGUE:

The Best Is Yet To Come!

By now, you've been barraged with information about FMS. You've also been told that it's not curable, and asked to continue to fight it as a battle that you can win. If there's one thing you must not give up, it is your positive attitude toward life. It's still worth living, and you can live an improved quality of life by learning to manage FMS instead of being controlled by it. I hope that reading this book as helped you to realize that truth.

Don't feel as if you must try everything at once in terms of the advice offered in these pages. In fact, you'll be better off if you don't. Start with you biggest thing to overcome and then work on that. Keep working on it until you have conquered it, and then move on to another area.

It's important that you get involved in the lives of others. Look around and search out a person who is in need of someone just like you to love and help them. You will notice at as you take your mind off your own problems and turn it toward others, your problems will begin mysteriously to appear smaller.

Search out a good FMS support group. But don't go to meetings and get caught up in the "poor old me pity parties." Find constructive ways to help others who are also afflicted with FMS, and share each other's victories.

More than any thing else, stick to it. You're going to need tenacity. Hold onto the hope that will put you into a bright future. Yes, you still have

one. God is not through with you!   You still have a
bright tomorrow…a life filled with laughter, hope,
health and promise…just wait and see.

Dr. Tim Weir

About The Author

Dr. Tim Weir is one of an emerging and new breed of cutting edge health care professionals who has dedicated his life to the healing of persons. You can't be around him for any length of time and not sense his deep commitment to seeing people med whole and having a richer and fuller total life experience. His years in the practice of healthcare have afforded him the opportunity to touch thousands of live and get the heart and soul of assisting individuals in cooperating with their bodies and attaining a greater degree of health and well being. He has had first hand experience with the sufferers of this strange condition and has seen the devastation it creates. In an effort to alleviate and ease the pain he has made room in his life to discover the missing pieces between what has been known and what has been unknown about this medical challenge.

You can listen to him on the daily syndicated radio show, Power Living Minute or listen to him on the downloadable podcast, Power Living Podcast. Don't expect it to be serious…his program was removed from one radio station for him saying, "pee-pee."

THE FIRST CHOICE LIFE SHOW
This 30 minute weekly television show is Dr. Weir's newest outreach. It is 30 minutes of inspiring, uplifting, practical information. Check our website to find a station near you. www.TheFirstChoiceLife.com. If you haven't found it…call your local stations and ask them why they don't have it on there!

Ordering Books and Supplements

Buy several of these books and hand them out to people you hang around. This will help them understand you a little better!
To order books and supplements, go to
www.The FirstChoiceLife.com

You can write Dr. Weir directly at:

Dr. Tim Weir
4109 Wake Forest Rd.
Suite 100
Raleigh, NC 27609

If you are in the Raleigh area, you can sometimes find Dr. Weir at the clinic. Call ahead of time if you are looking to talk to him!